Faith

VS. WEIGHT

Faith

VS. WEIGHT

Magnifying the Glory of God by Reclaiming Your Energy to Serve the Kingdom

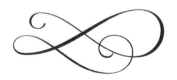

Maria V. Bower, MBA, NASM-CPT

DISCLAIMER

Seek a physician's approval before starting any weight loss or exercise program.

FAITH VS. WEIGHT is not a substitute for medical supervision. Annual physicals are an important part of preventative health and can weed out medical issues that may affect weight management. Whether or not you are currently on medications causing you to gain or retain weight, the biblical lessons in this book will inspire you to make better choices! Your body needs appropriate nutrition and exercise in order for it to function optimally, whether it is running a race, recovering from an illness, or managing a disease. The nutrition and exercise principles presented in this book are purposefully meant to complement your physician's care, not replace it. Average clients lose one to two pounds per week. Results will vary.

The author has made every effort to ensure the accuracy of the information within this book was correct at time of publication. The author does not assume and hereby disclaims any liability to any party for any loss, damage, or disruption caused by errors or omissions, whether such errors or omissions result from accident, negligence, or any other cause. Some names and identifying details have been changed to protect the privacy of individuals.

This book is designed to provide helpful information and inspiration to readers. This book is not meant to be used, nor should it be used, to diagnose or treat any medical condition. For diagnosis or treatment of any medical problem, consult your physician. The publisher and author are not responsible for any specific health or allergy needs that may require medical supervision and are not liable for any

to my Mother

Thank you for always being
my number one fan.

CONTENTS

Acknowledgments xi

Author's Note xv

How to Use This Book 1

What Is FAITH VS. WEIGHT? 5

Preface 11

Introduction 17

Week One: Prudence 35

Week Two: Temperance 81

Week Three: Faith 123

Week Four: Justice 171

Week Five: Perseverance 205

Week Six: Hope 241

Week Seven: Love 279

Conclusion 321

Afterword 325

Prayer for Salvation 331

Appendix: The FAITH VS. WEIGHT Diet

    Eating Timing and Tips 334

    Breakfast/Snack Chart 338

    Lunch/Dinner Chart 340

    Restaurant Guide 342

    Restaurant Options 348

    Testimonials 355

    A Day in the Life of a Diabetic Q&A 361

About the Author 363

Acknowledgments

I thank my eternal Father in heaven for saving my life: past, present, and future. His unending love, guiding me each step along the way, has granted this sinner the privilege to serve His kingdom. Without His love, there would be no one to thank. Because of His love, there are too many to thank, but I will do the best I can. How can I ever be thankful enough?

To My Church Family

I thank Prestonwood Baptist Church (PBC), led by Dr. Jack Graham, for the opportunity to learn the entire Bible, not just the parts I wanted to hear. You have facilitated an environment that will echo the Word of God throughout eternity by encouraging church staff and members to use their gifts for His glory. Our family has steadily grown closer to the Lord Jesus Christ as a result of the Holy Spirit working through you and Dr. Jarett Stephens.

Chrissie Dunham of PBC Women's Ministry, there are no words to describe your zeal for the kingdom. Thank you for giving me an invitation to Eternal Life, illuminating the Word of God, and providing an outlet to share it through FAITH VS. WEIGHT. As for my other sister in Christ, Suzy Bastian, please know how grateful I am for your extraordinary teaching, love, and support, forever influencing the course of my family's destiny. The women of Prestonwood and their families are blessed beyond measure to have you two as leaders who continue to spread the Gospel, whatever the cost. Thank you, Laura Howell, for sharing your innumerable gifts and for humbly keeping us all on track!

I also want to thank Prestonwood Sports Organization (PSO) for the opportunity to share the Good News through fitness. I couldn't have done it without the welcoming kindred spirit of Toby Graham and my adopted mentor,

Lee Truax. The ongoing support of each PSO staff member, including Tony Lewandowski, Gayle Mixon, and Brian Bennett has been unwavering.

I cannot list everyone in the Prestonwood community that has inspired, encouraged, supported, and loved me and my family through this process. However, I thank God for each one of you, as you represent the body of Christ, especially the Mims-Cross, Von-Tress, Lineberger, Eubanks, and Colan families. To the Panetti and Snyder families, your friendship, love, and support, personally and through your Sunday School teaching, have been a beacon throughout this process.

Thank you, Molly Bastian Coulter, for taking the time to get that perfect shot. You are a gifted photographer!

To My Editors

Hailee Willhite, you are as insightful as you are kind and beautiful. Thank you for giving me the confidence to move forward as my dear friend and biblical editor. Many clients tell me they hear my voice in their head, just as I heard yours while I was writing this book. A special thank you to Chris for whatever time this took away from your family!

Linda Yawn, I praise God for your daughter, Marya Lewis, and for putting the two of us together! Thank you for taking my rough draft and effectively transforming it. I could have looked for years and not found anyone as remotely dedicated to putting in the passion and commitment that you selflessly poured into this book. You were a heaven-sent answer to prayer. Thank you for taking the time to condense, edit, and rewrite my work! I tried to incorporate as many of your expert suggestions as I could, but discovered I am a serious "word hoarder" in the process!

To My Clients

Each of you has taught me a thing or two about perseverance, love, and faith. You have helped develop a program that will positively impact families you may never meet. I am eternally grateful for your selfless honesty throughout this process! To my faithful morning exercisers, you made my days brighter as we shared our joys and heartbreak, all while praising the Lord and getting in a good workout. To my past and present clients who have become steadfast friends, thank you for revealing my calling: Pat King, Rhonda James, Brianna Hinojosa-Smith, Tia Dali, Kippie Masepohl, Keri Muir, Nesa Anders, Christie Sheedy, Gwen Kelley, Sarah Eubanks, Jamie Windle, Suzette Snyder, Jess Amason, Linda Rodgers, Beth Criner, Jane Mixdorf, Linda Overstreet, and my dear friend Stacie Allen.

To My Extended Family

Thank you for loving my family through good times and bad. To the Galatolie family, you made all the difference. Know that you are loved. To Charlotte Sueverkruebbe, I couldn't have done this without you. Thank you for your flexibility and servant spirit!

To My Family

To my number one fan, my Mother, Roseanne Volpe, thank you for your prayers, encouragement, and love. Your enthusiasm for this book has blessed me in more ways than you can imagine. Frank, Joelle, and the Volpe Den, thank you for being an example of a family rooted in Christ. To the Romance/Cocomello family, thank you for your ongoing love and support. Thanks also go to John Corvo for checking in throughout this process. Gina Savini, I would have to say you are as good as family at this point.

To Sarah and Bill Bower, how can I ever thank you for raising such an amazing man of God? I am so blessed to be a part of a family who impacts so many others through faithful acts of generosity, kindness, and love. You both do an untold number of small acts with great love! To Jeff, Michelle, and your families, thank you for your continued support, encouragement, and love throughout this journey.

To Matthew and Benjamin, what an unparalleled gift it is to be your mother! I am so proud of each of you and your commitment to excellence but most importantly for your love of the Lord and your neighbor. Thank you for sharing the Word of God with me while also challenging me to keep up!

Benjamin, you have an exuberant and generous heart with an intellect to match. You are always ready to encourage someone in the classroom or on the mission field through your activities that are too long to list! You make me a better person by reminding me to be sensitive to the needs of others.

Matthew, your strength and compassion come through, whether I see you holding the door for an injured classmate, teaching piano, or playing soccer. Your intelligence, perseverance, and attention to detail are admirable. I can't wait to see the plans the Lord has for you and your brother.

To My Favorite Person

Mark, if I had my life to live over again, "I'd find you sooner so I could love you longer." Thank you for being even better than the person I thought you were, which was pretty hard to beat. The Lord truly blessed me with a "prince among men" when he gave me you as my husband.

To my Father, who is now able to see Jesus face-to-face, I don't know if I ever had the chance to tell you what Mark told me after he met you ... "There is a lot of Daddy in you." Thank you for leaving me your best for His glory.

Finally, a special thank you to the prior leadership team of the Coppell Family YMCA. Because of the guidance and support of Gayle Westapher and Gina Boznak, FAITH VS. WEIGHT became a reality. Tia Dali, this book was written because of you.

Author's Note

Wake up, sleeper, rise from the dead, and Christ will shine on you.
—Ephesians 5:14 (NIV)

My dear friend, it's not about your thighs. It's about your "why." Why do you want to lose weight in the first place? Every day, more and more of us are succumbing to a zombie-like existence, heading aimlessly toward our demise. This is because many of us have not identified a big enough reason why. We may go on another diet or try a new exercise class for a week or a month, but nothing sticks. Either we try something unsustainable, or we give up, repeating this pattern over and over. We rarely commit long-term to the basics of healthy eating and exercise because it takes commitment, and our why is just not worth it. Although we spend significant amounts of time and money on vanity, this does not seem to be a big enough reason either. Apparently, neither is fear, since most people do not make radical lifestyle changes even after their doctor delivers the bad news. The only reason big enough to inspire you to eat healthy and exercise over the long haul is *love*.

Although both losing weight and gaining energy top most people's New Year's resolution lists year after year, we eat and exercise as if both were our last priority. It's as if we know we should want a healthier life, but the effort is just not worth it. As a friend once said, "I am willing to try anything in order to lose weight … except a healthy diet and exercise." We had a good laugh, but she nailed it when it comes to describing our society as a whole. We throw money at the problem, starting with the least to most expensive fix, including caffeine, drugs, hormones, and even surgery, but we are either not willing to work at it, or we overdo it. Unfortunately, since most people are chasing after the wrong why, for the wrong reasons, we wind up also chasing after the wrong solutions, never breaking free from *weight loss groundhog day*.

Instead, how different would your choices be if you looked at food as either creating energy or draining it, because that is exactly what it is doing! You will never make progress with your health until you realize how your choices affect your energy and how your lack of energy ultimately limits your choices. Unless you make the connection that how you treat your body directly affects what you can expect from it, you will never win. If you are not convinced reclaiming your energy in order to more fully love yourself, your family, and your community in Jesus's name is far greater than any perceived sacrifice, you will never commit long-term to a healthy eating and exercise plan.

What if you looked at having more energy as a chance to better fulfill your God-given destiny? What if you realized having more energy is not just a nice perk but necessary to equip you to achieve what He is calling you to do? It's about having enough energy to love. It's about swimming with your kids instead of worrying about how you look in a bathing suit. It may be about serving in your career, whether it's in business, education, or public office. It's all ultimately about serving with love, and serving takes energy.

There may be an important assignment God is calling you to do, but you are just too maxed out and distracted by the end of the day to even hear His call on your life because of a junk food coma. More and more people are in this boat. Instead of wasting time on guilt, a luxury we can no longer afford, it's time to wake up. The sugar highs are not worth the physical, emotional, and spiritual lows. The kingdom of God needs you today, not Monday, when you start your next diet! Jesus did not die on the cross for you or I to half-heartedly crawl through another workweek. He came to give abundant life through His grace so we not only have enough energy for what He calls us to do but also to make a difference in the lives He has given us the opportunity to serve.

If you are not more excited about your why, instead of whatever junk is in front of you, then you will not walk away from it. This is the real reason, besides a diet being unsustainable, why many fail in their efforts or gain the weight back. Most people are just not excited about their potential to magnify God's glory, because they have no idea what they are missing. Most of the time, we don't even realize we are missing out on anything other than the inconvenient expense of having to buy new clothes or having to take meds. Meanwhile, life is passing us by one junk food coma at a time. It's not until we recognize something is stealing our joy that we start looking for a scapegoat. Even then, we are not fully aware of what is going on because we blame our lack of energy on aging or a host of other things instead of what we are putting in our mouths. Over time, there are consequences. We wind up rendered ineffective in fulfilling our mission on a small or epic scale. We are asleep at the wheel. Not only are we uninspired, we are not even awake.

This does not need to be your fate! Excess weight is a problem just like any other, and the tools taught here to manage this problem will spill over into other areas of your life. Like all other distractions from the devil, it is a problem that is stealing your energy from serving God, making you miserable in the process. It is time to reclaim your energy for His glory to serve His kingdom with love. This epidemic no longer needs to stop you and your family from reaching your full potential in Christ. There is too much at stake. The life saved may be your own, but it will hopefully not be the only one.

"Wake up, sleeper," while it is still today, because today is all that you and I have got.

So whether you
eat or drink or whatever you do,
do it all for the glory of God.

—1 Corinthians 10:31 (NIV)

How to Use This Book

This book's purpose is to inspire, illuminate, and transform. First we must inspire a call to action. Enough is enough. If the reason we want to lose weight isn't big enough, we will not succeed. Next we have to illuminate or expose the real problem, which is a faulty mind-set coupled with years of nutrition misinformation. We need a plan that makes sense. We need to know what to do. Finally, we will transform our souls, minds, and ultimately our bodies through this process. We need to know how to do this.

Inspiration (Why)

Question: Why do I want to do this?

Answer: To glorify God.

A lack of inspiration is the number one reason most people are not healthy. We are uninspired because we do not realize our sole purpose is to glorify God. There is no greater purpose than that! Once this sinks in, we need to answer, "What does glorifying God look like in my life?" In order to focus our efforts, we will develop a strategic plan to reclaim our energy and fulfill our calling.

Illumination (What)

Question: Now that we are inspired, what do we need to do in order to succeed?

Answer: Come up with a realistic plan.

We are often unrealistic in our planning or lack of planning partly because we do not know what to do regarding diet and exercise. Usually, when it comes to timing, we want results yesterday. This doesn't mean our strategic outlook is unrealistic, but our timeline or plans often are. Most people do things every day they believe are helping them lose weight, which are instead packing on the pounds. This is where we need to be educated or illuminated. Included in this book is a nutrition and fitness plan that has helped many of my clients to lose and maintain their weight loss. Food timing and planning are included. This plan does not eliminate any food groups. We address why we should adopt a balanced nutrition and exercise plan instead of a sensational quick fix. We also specify best exercises according to body type and weight loss in general. It is not necessary to kill yourself in order to lose weight.

TRANSFORMATION (HOW)

Question: How does this work in our lives with our crazy schedules?

Answer: We walk with the Lord!

Even if we have a sound strategic outlook backed by a realistic plan, we must realize this is a journey that we cannot do alone. This is the third reason many fail at their attempts. We need to learn how to go the distance. Although the first few weeks have an emphasis on nutrition, while the latter weeks dive into movement, every week is designed to strengthen our faith. In the "Change Your Life" section, we receive specific guidelines and suggestions on how improve in all three areas. This is why the program takes seven weeks. In order to have new life, old habits need to die to make room for new ones.

PUTTING IT ALL TOGETHER

Each chapter is based on one of the seven virtues, which are frequently discussed throughout the Bible. These virtues will act as a road map wisely guiding us on our weight-loss journey. Four of the seven virtues (prudence, temperance, justice, and perseverance) are traced back to Greek philosophy, and the remaining three to the Judeo-Christian tradition (faith, hope, and love). Each chapter applies one of the virtues to weight management in the following format:

- Love the Lord Your God
- Change Your Brain
- Eat for Energy
- Make Your Move
- Take a Stand
- Love Your Neighbor
- Change Your Life

As we follow this format, we will gently incorporate healthy lifestyle changes without torturing ourselves or going through total withdrawal. At least one treat is allowed every day during this process as we determine what does and does not work. Everyone is different, so no two plans will look alike.

WARNING: DIET ALONE WILL NOT CHANGE YOUR BEHAVIOR

These virtues are synergistic and work best if they are applied together. Skipping straight to the diet is going to eventually lead you right back to where you started. Realize this program exists for a reason. Everyone is excited about a new diet in the beginning. Then old behaviors and doubts start to surface by week two or three. Our program differs from others since we tackle recurring issues that have held us back. Our hearts, minds, and bodies will change as we take each week to gain momentum and overcome recurring strongholds.

WARNING: PUT YOUR OXYGEN MASK ON FIRST

Hold off trying to fix others, including family, if they are not excited to participate. You may want to limit talking about the fact that you are making healthy lifestyle changes to only the most supportive members. Many have struggled with changing their own behavior and have become cynical. They may question your chances for success or project on you the fate they suffered, which is distracting and discouraging. Skip the negativity. Misery loves company, and this is not the company you want to keep.

The best way to help others reclaim their energy is by first reclaiming your own. It is not until the very last week (week seven) of the transformation that we include others in the program who either want to be included or for whom we can serve as an example. Our success can inspire others, including our kids. There are different strategies for different situations.

If you want to help others, you must put your oxygen mask on first. Once you reach your goal, you can shout it from the rooftops, but this will not be necessary since everyone will see your results firsthand and inquire how you accomplished such a feat.

Warning: This Is A Seven Week Program

This is not a quick fix. To best prepare, continue reading until you have completed the introduction. At that point you are ready to begin! Starting with week one, only read one chapter at a time. Give yourself a full week to absorb each chapter. It takes time to change lifelong habits, but it's worth it!

What Is
FAITH VS. WEIGHT?

MISSION STATEMENT: MAGNIFYING THE GLORY OF GOD BY RECLAIMING YOUR ENERGY TO SERVE THE KINGDOM!

FAITH VS. WEIGHT (FVW) is a seven-week program that applies biblical wisdom to the chaotic world of weight management. Instead of starving one minute and binging the next, we are biblically inspired to attain and maintain our personal nutrition and fitness victories. Each week inspires increased faith in the Lord Jesus Christ while also providing strategies geared toward effective health and weight management. The faith and the weight parts of this program are inseparable. Progress in one area affects progress in the other. Although many participants have tried every diet under the sun and were already burned out from various false starts, this program was their breakthrough, whether they had previously tried other faith-based programs or not.

As a prior US Navy health care administrator and current certified personal trainer, I found the one thing missing from most weight-loss programs was wisdom. Common sense did not seem to prevail when it came to long-term weight management. In order to provide a program based on wisdom, I went to the source. The same biblical wisdom applies today as it did two thousand years ago. In our world of overbooked schedules, executive leadership positions, fast food, delayed flights, sick kids, birthday parties, shared-custody agreements, handicaps, chronic diseases, demanding work schedules, international travel, carpools, playdates, and late-night client dinners, we need wisdom now more than ever!

From a practical standpoint, this program can be as simple or as fancy as you like. If you hate cooking, fear not because there are zero-cook options for those who cannot handle boiling water. The other good news is you will not give up any food groups (unless you want to), buy any magic potions or pills, or weigh yourself every day—or at all. And you do not need to be a shut-in. This program teaches you how to eat in restaurants and airports and at formal functions as well as how to navigate kids' (or grandkids') birthday parties.

FVW is a lifestyle. No one is starving, counting calories, or doing Ironman triathlons (unless they want to), and no one is eating the same food repetitively. It is designed for real people and delivers real results. Initially designed for group settings, it has also been successfully implemented by individuals, couples, and families. However, when changing behavior, the power of a group has been demonstrated repeatedly. Supportive group environments have been successful in changing habits for alcoholics and drug addicts for decades, in both inpatient and outpatient settings. People struggling with overeating can only benefit from what members of these groups have already learned the hard way: it's easier not to go it alone. My prayer is for this program to be used within a group for support and fellowship. (Yes, two or more count.) However, this program has been absolutely successful with individuals as well. Do what works for you.

FVW was developed for the women of the Coppell Family YMCA in Coppell, Texas, and is currently being offered through the Women's Ministry of Prestonwood Baptist Church in Plano, Texas.

Most of my clients were in good shape before they woke up a few years later realizing their ten extra pounds had turned into twenty, thirty, or more. Many were in better shape than I was as a kid. Whatever stage you are in now, it is not permanent. It is only hopeless for those who have given up hope. Perhaps this is the reason Jesus centered most of his teaching on faith.

> *Now faith is confidence in what we hope for and assurance about what we do not see.*
>
> *—Hebrews 11:1 (NIV)*

Changing from a mind-set of defeat to victory requires a leap of faith. However, once you have faith, the rest will come naturally. This program works on strengthening your faith. The diet is the easy part. Whether you spend your time in airports or sitting in the carpool line day after day while taking care of the most important people in your life, we coax the weight off while you live one day at a time.

A lack of faith when it comes to improving our diets has caused many to settle. Unfortunately, you may conclude that as long as you are doing better than your next-door neighbor, you are fine. Although chronic conditions seem to come out of nowhere when we receive an unsavory diagnosis, most do not appear overnight. You may blame aging for a lack of energy and chronic conditions, but aging is only part of this equation—and less than most people want to admit. Our current state of health is a result of our choices over time, and our choices are greatly affected by our beliefs.

Many people believe they are not strong enough to make better choices on a consistent basis. Are you one of them? If so, you may be right about not being strong enough. If you think you are unable to make the necessary lifestyle changes on your own, you are correct. Congratulations! You are the winner! You cannot do this on your own. Does this mean you are out of options? Nope. You can choose to ask God to give you the strength to change your habits one day at a time. He can do the heavy lifting.

Although you may be a diet veteran, you may or may not have had prior experience as a thin person. Everyone must start somewhere, so why not here? You may think everyone else has a better chance than you, especially your neighbor down the street. She must have been born that way. She loves to exercise and eat broccoli. Some people think I was born that way. I was actually nicknamed Broccoli in a parenting class because I suggested going for a bike ride with our kids instead of going to eat doughnuts. No one called me Broccoli growing up. Quite the contrary, I never experienced a family bike ride as a child. Most of my meals were larger servings than I needed. Growing up in an abusive household, food was my comfort. It was not until a few years after my parents divorced that I eventually was able to eat healthier. As for exercise, I never ran around the block or played a sport. I was considered too fat for anyone to want me on her team.

By today's standards, I would have been considered pleasantly plump, but back then, I was considered just plain fat. That's because the standards we judge weight by have gotten a lot looser. If you have been called fat, you are in good company! So what happened? Did my metabolism get faster? Did I take weight-loss supplements? Did I have a killer trainer? Well, no. Although I did become a trainer, that is not what brought me victory. It is written that if you believe Jesus is the Son of God, you have already overcome. My victory comes from the Lord Jesus Christ. So does yours.

> *Who is it that overcomes the world? Only the one who believes that Jesus is the Son of God.*
>
> *—1 John 5:5 (NIV)*

As a child, I was teased for being fat, so I know how painful it can be. Haven't we wasted enough tears on being fat? It doesn't really matter what anyone else thinks. All that matters is that you have the energy and the agility to be the best you can be to answer your calling. Just know that even with injuries, surgeries, relocations, disease, accidents, and aging, not only do you not need to gain weight, but you can also lose whatever excess you are carrying. This is the case even if you have "fat" genes. This also applies to pregnancies, including those surprises arriving later in life than expected.

Today, it requires a daily commitment, but I have victory in Christ. Healthy lifestyle choices have become a habit. I no longer make New Year's resolutions about fitness or diet because I am already happy with my fitness level and diet. This is the goal I have for all of my clients. Although it took me almost fifty years to get here, I can save you the time. As a personal trainer certified through the National Academy of Sports Medicine (NASM) who specializes in weight loss, fitness nutrition, women's fitness, group fitness, and behavioral change, I am blessed to guide my clients and their families to victory. This book will help you to achieve the same.

Make Your Faith a Reality

People put their faith in a lot of different things. Some people will only put their faith in the diet part of this program. That is the wrong approach. The faith this book refers to is in the Lord Jesus Christ alone. Faith is the difference between victory and defeat for your weight-loss miracle. You cannot succeed without it. Whether you are just starting out in your faith journey or are a church leader, you haven't come this far to stunt your growth. The rest of this plan shows veterans as well as new believers practical ways to connect with the Almighty regarding your health. Start with what works for you. It's time to apply your faith to your weight.

Preface

I have set before you life and death, blessings and curses. Now choose life, so that you and your children may live.

—Deuteronomy 30:19 (NIV)

As a health and wellness coach and former health care administrator for the US Navy, I am concerned about our health as a nation. In the United States, before we even begin to think about foreign enemies, we must first consider our own worst domestic enemy. Our obesity epidemic reminds me of one of Khrushchev's quotes: "We won't have to fight you ... until you'll fall like overripe fruit into our hands." Although he was referring to our economy, I think about it in terms of our nation's health. Other countries can sit back and watch our demise. It is like the fall of the Roman Empire. For the first time, we are struggling to find recruits for our military who meet entry-level weight standards.

Income level, demographics, education, and age do not seem to matter. I have observed situations where healthy, unprocessed food was fresh and plentiful, yet people still chose the unhealthy, overly processed options. Those with higher income levels may have picked fancier processed foods, but they are still far from what nature intended. For most people living in developed countries, this has less to do with availability and more to do with priorities. Since we put our money where our mouth is, we are creating an atmosphere that is hostile to our health. This is a war we have brought upon ourselves.

There are two questions that need to be answered when prioritizing your health.

1) What reward am I seeking? (Do I want to reclaim my energy to glorify God and serve His kingdom, or would I rather have the life sucked out of me while I blame my lack of energy and excess weight on everything and everybody else?)

You might say the reward you are seeking is improved health and energy. Yet, for many, this is not the reward they are pursuing on a daily basis. When it comes to eating, most are looking for immediate gratification, which usually entails sugar and unhealthy fats. Because so many options overstimulate your palate, you get a heightened sense of reward, and you just keep eating. You are chasing the wrong reward.

What if your heart could convince your brain to crave a different reward? Mine has, as is the case with many of my clients. We didn't start out this way, but through Jesus Christ, we now have our eyes fixed on a different prize because we have our eyes on Jesus. The decision was made long before we ever picked up the second piece of birthday cake or skipped the gym again. Instead, we are reclaiming our energy to glorify God. This reward has become our priority! We are human beings and fail at it. However, we have the gift of grace, and this gift allows us to get back in the race. Once you get started, remember you are only one meal or walk away from getting back on track when you veer off the path.

> *I press toward the goal for the prize of the upward call of God in Christ Jesus.*
>
> *—Philippians 3:14 (NKJV)*

2) How am I going to claim this reward? (Is what I am about to eat, drink, or do going to give me more energy to glorify God or is it going to suck the life right out of me?)

In our country, if you have access to food, you are most likely sugar addicted. Although slaying the sugar dragon is a critical part of this plan, it does not necessarily mean you will never have sugar again. It does mean you need to get your blood sugar under control. The better control you have, the better chance of your losing weight. Many of my clients are either ashamed of or in denial about their being sugar addicted. Once the realization hits, they feel either relieved or depressed. There is nothing wrong with them or you. Unless you are buying real food in its original state, you can bet sugar has been added. I rarely meet someone who has not had a problem with sugar, salt, or fatty meats. Since the human body was not designed for starvation, we consume products offering short-term relief regardless of their potential for long-term damage.

To combat this, we have to fix our stomachs while we fix our heads. Each week, you will gain confidence as you are given specific guidelines to work your plan. We are dealing with physiological as well as psychological issues. It is easiest to deal with physiology! To get blood sugar to a more manageable state, we have to nourish our body with real food at the right times so we do not fall victim to the wrong choices. Whether we are hungry with real hunger or false hunger, triggered by sugar highs and lows, sugar is waving the quick energy flag, and we are dealing with physiological urges that go beyond our will power. The only successful way to satisfy these urges is to eat real balanced food at regular intervals before we are desperate for the processed options. Because processed foods rarely satisfy, they lead to overeating. As one of my diabetic clients shared in class, "Sugar craves sugar." And I might add: fake sugars crave sugar! For many people, carbs crave carbs, even the good ones, depending on how your body handles them. This does not mean we will never have sugar or quality carbs again, but timing and amounts are important. We have to eat a breakfast that balances our blood sugar before we are in front of the box of doughnuts in the office break room or teachers' lounge. A smoothie advertising that it balances blood sugar, containing a paragraph of ingredients, sets most people up for failure. Instead, this plan has delicious smoothie options that you can make at home with three real ingredients that take only five minutes to prepare.

Food is meant to satisfy hunger, not create it. People are either eating what they think is a healthy breakfast, making their hunger worse later in the day, or they are not eating breakfast at all because they binged on junk food the night before, repeating the same process. Breakfast really is the most important meal of the day.

There are two reasons people say they are always hungry. The first reason is most are not getting the right ratios of protein, fat, and carbohydrates to satisfy real hunger at regular intervals. The second reason, amplifying the first problem, is most are on a sugar roller coaster, creating false hunger. To get off this ride, we must prioritize the right food combinations (protein, fat, and carbohydrate ratios) at the right time in order to decrease, instead of increase, cravings. We will learn simple ways to do this. This needs to happen before the cookie, bagel, or doughnut tempts us.

Many are being robbed of a healthy life, pulling their own trigger. The more sugar and processed foods we eat, the more we crave, and these choices add up over time. The reason real food doesn't taste good to us any more is because we crave what we eat. When I hear someone does not like vegetables, I believe them. We have trained our palates to like only processed foods. However, the Bible does not mention anyone starving to death due to a lack of processed foods. Instead, it cautions us to not overdo sweets or meats. No matter who you are, you can eat healthy and enjoy it! God actually knew what He was doing when He spoke vegetation into existence and told us it was food. Eating meat came after that. What do you think Noah ate after the flood?

Unfortunately, in our society, you cannot just show up and assume there will be healthy options. Instead, you must plan ahead and have the right strategy in place. The good news is there is a lot you can do that requires minimal effort! Whether your personality type is one who jumps in and makes immediate dietary changes or implements them more slowly, working on one meal at a time, victory is ultimately yours if you persevere. Just like a boxer, you may have to go several rounds, but it's worth it. A healthy diet is a reward, not a sacrifice, because it supplies energy instead of draining it. Although victory in this area is its own reward, the potential impact you can have when you reclaim your energy, fulfilling your potential for God's glory, is far greater!

You might have gone from starving one minute to binging the next as you skipped from one diet to another. Many assume that a lack of making healthy choices equals a lack of willpower or self-discipline. I disagree. I know many disciplined individuals who struggle with their weight. It is a lack of being in tune with why you want to live a healthy lifestyle and choosing the right diet and exercise plan to get you there. When the word *diet* is used with regard to FVW, I am not talking deprivation but rather increased vitality. If we regularly ate a diet of real food, balancing our portions, with a small dessert after dinner, while remaining moderately active, we would be just fine. Many cultures around the world do this, and they are not obese because they stick to their traditional diet. Instead, we are having dessert all day, every day, starting with breakfast.

Before insisting you are not in this category, I challenge you to see if you reach the same conclusion after reading this book. Because of the media hype surrounding certain food products, you may be eating things you believe are healthier than real food, cheating both yourself and your children. I am not writing this to make you feel guilty. My hope is to awaken in you a different type of hunger. The Lord Jesus Christ came to give you "fullness of life" in all areas, including your health. It's time to reclaim it.

Beloved, I pray that in all respects you may prosper and be in good health, just as your soul prospers.

—3 John 1:2 (NASB)

Introduction

Do you want to be healed? — Will & desire

—*John 5:6 (MEV)*

This is what Jesus asked an invalid in Jerusalem near a pool called Bethesda where the sick, lame, blind, and paralyzed would lie day after day, year after year, hoping for a miracle. An angel would come and stir the water. If you wanted to be healed, you had to get in the pool immediately after the angel stirred the water, or you were out of luck. Jesus knew the man who was lying there had been suffering for thirty-eight years. He had spent a lifetime within sitting distance of his miracle but was not even able to get a toe in.

This passage reminds me of our obesity epidemic since we have at our fingertips access to world-class preventative health, nutrition, fitness equipment, trainers, gyms, apps, and gadgets, yet we never quite seem to attain or maintain our weight-loss miracle. So the question remains ...

"Do you want to be healed?"

Why wouldn't the invalid want to be healthy? Didn't God know this man wanted to be healthy his whole life? Doesn't God know we *all* want to be healed? Who wants to be an invalid?

I was contemplating this verse, which I often refer to when teaching FAITH VS. WEIGHT, after an awe-inspiring visit to the Museum of the Bible in Washington, DC. Our flight was full, with passengers traveling to Dallas/ Fort Worth who happened to be enjoying a chocolate Danish or two. These passengers were just eating the way most people eat on vacation. Some were having a second glass of wine. It was 10:00 a.m. Unfortunately, as a health and wellness coach, I know that many will later tell themselves they have fat genes (which may be true) and that they are doomed to be overweight (which is not true) when their pants feel tight.

You were bought with a price; do not become slaves.

—1 Corinthians 7:23 (NIV)

Although there were healthier options available, most of the passengers went for the chocolate Danish. Even with choices, most Americans would choose the chocolate Danish. Misdiagnosing our real problem, we decide to blame our obesity epidemic on something or somebody else. If we only had the right metabolism, genes, schedule, husband, willpower, personal chef, celebrity trainer, or Bethesda angel, we would not have a weight problem. Just like the invalid who believed the answer to his problem was just beyond his grasp, we often believe our weight-loss victory is just beyond our reach as well. Because of these lies, we are defeated before we even begin. We are chasing after the wrong solutions because we are unable to admit what our real problem is. The above verse talks about becoming a slave to other human beings. Instead, we have become slaves to our appetites.

Although we want to be healed, we make excuses. Satan's entire purpose is "to steal and kill and destroy" —John 10:10 (NIV). So he is quick to provide us with a never-ending list. With substance-abuse issues, including food, the supposed power an inanimate object holds over us is just another one of his lies. Yet many of us substitute his lies for our truth, robbing God of His glory. Rather than a guilt trip, this is meant to set you free. Most of us either have no idea we are enslaved by our food choices or we feel guilty about it. You can continue to believe the lie that you will remain a slave to an inanimate substance or you can fight back with the Word of God. There is no other alternative. Whether your weakness is media, alcohol, drugs, porn, or food, Satan will do whatever he can to drown you in your substance of choice, especially at your weakest moments. He will either distort your reality by tricking you into thinking your particular problem is too big for God to solve, or even better, he will convince you that you are still in control, when in reality you are enslaved. If we do finally realize we have a problem, we assume it is our fault because we are weak, or we blame something or someone else. It doesn't matter which lie we choose to believe, either way we are defeated. Just like the invalid, we make excuses.

"I have no one to help me into the pool when the water is stirred. While I am trying to get in, someone else goes down ahead of me."

—*John 5:7 (NIV)*   What's your excuse?

Getting straight to the point, Jesus replied, "Get up! Pick up your mat and walk." —John 5:8 (NIV). It almost seems like Jesus was telling him to wake up. You are not getting any younger.

MIRACULOUS CUSTOMER SERVICE

Remove far from me falsehood and lies. Give me neither poverty nor riches. Feed me with the food that is needful for me.

—*Proverbs 30:8 (WEB)*

When the invalid told Jesus, "Someone else goes down ahead of me," not only was he blaming others, but it also sounds like he believed miracles were for everybody but him. Likewise, Satan wants to convince you that this is as good as it gets—or even better, that God has forgotten you. Did you know that believing your problem is beyond God's healing power is a type of vanity?

Faith is trusting God to take care of all of our needs. He defines our needs differently than we do. We think our needs are too big for God to satisfy because we confuse wants with needs. We want to get rid of the weight, but we don't want to be bothered with the faith. Satan will take a want and convince us it is a need. This causes doubt as to whether or not God will ever satisfy any of our needs. Many people assuage this uneasiness with food. Besides, do we really have a guarantee God will take care of all of our needs? The answer is yes. This is one of the ways He manifests His glory.

> *My God will supply every need of yours according to his riches in glory*
> *in Christ Jesus.*
>
> —*Philippians 4:19 (WEB)*

When we assume God cannot help us with our needs, we are tying His hands and withholding His glory. We do this by doubting Him. I have actually heard clients say, "Maybe I am just meant to be fat." Since we are not God, we are clearly better off not jumping to that conclusion, or we may be right.

> *So tell them, "As surely as I live, declares the LORD, I will do to you*
> *the very thing I heard you say."*
>
> —*Numbers 14:28 (NIV)*

Since He is listening, you are clearly better off praising Him than accusing. The Bible tells us we need to take care of our bodies. If you are going to blame God for having a slow metabolism, you should also admit He has provided healthy food and plenty of opportunities for exercise as well. A slow metabolism does not mean God is unable to help you take care of your body. As an eleven-year-old child weighing a hundred pounds in fifth grade, I never imagined that someday I would be considered fit. Recently, my metabolism was tested, and my metabolism is faster than most people my age and younger. The logical way to explain this is as a child I had more fat than muscle (compared to other fifth graders). I now have more muscle than fat (compared to other fifty-two-year-olds). I was also much slower than most fifth graders and did not participate in any sports. Recently, I came home with a large plastic trophy, First Place, Women's Master Division, 5K. This would have been impossible without faith in the Lord.

> *"Not by might, nor by power, but by my Spirit."*
>
> —*Zechariah 4:6 (WEB)*

Faith allows God to manifest His glory, but first you have to identify the problem. Things like fat genes and slow metabolisms are not show-stoppers for God. Even with fat genes, you can have a faster metabolism and improve your level of fitness relative to your age group. Strength training, cardio, and the right type and amounts of food can increase your metabolism. Most people hear "faster metabolism" and immediately think they need to kill it at the gym. That mentality is what keeps us fat. A balanced approach to fitness and nutrition is what works over the long haul. You must apply His wisdom to this equation, not the quick fix or lies of the devil. It takes faith in order for God to manifest His glory. No faith equals no power.

> *Now to him who is able to do exceeding abundantly above all that we ask or think, according to the power that works in us.*
>
> *—Ephesians 3:20 (WEB)*

The "power that works in us" comes from God through Jesus Christ. This doesn't mean you are overweight because you lack faith in God, as you may be a person of great faith. However, in this area of your life, you may not have achieved victory. Even when medical issues have been ruled out, you still may not see your blind spots, but it doesn't mean they don't exist. This is why they are called blind spots. We all have them. You may feel as if you are doing everything right to maintain a healthy diet and exercise plan but are still struggling! It is common to do things that work for others but not for you. Stop worrying about everyone else. Pray for the veil to be lifted from your eyes to gain insight as to what works best for your body and your spirit. Both belong to God.

> *For you were bought with a price. Therefore glorify God in your body and in your spirit, which are God's.*
>
> *—1 Corinthians 6:20 (WEB)*

INVALID THINKING

Many people are slaves to their appetites. This is why diets don't work. People have asked me, "Can you skip the God part already and just give me the diet?" I previously gave people a cheat sheet version of the diet because I thought it would save time. Since most people do not stay committed to diets, this approach rarely worked. It just wasted more time. Many people lose weight on diets without a faith component attached, and you can also lose weight. However, if this has been a lifelong struggle for you, then you need more than a diet. You need the truth.

> *Guide me in your truth, and teach me, For you are the God of my salvation, I wait for you all day long.*
>
> *—Psalm 25:5 (WEB)*

That's because in many cases this is more of a faith problem than a weight problem. Beyond perceived needs created by the devil, you have valid needs. Many fill the valid need of hunger with the invalid choice of a candy bar, chips, or overdoing it with real food, which creates a vicious cycle. This may be out of carelessness, but if it happens more often than not, you have become a slave to your appetite. Continuous overeating of garbage is a symptom of a bigger problem. We doubt our innermost needs will ever be met, so we either give up on a healthy lifestyle or feel guilty about not pursuing one. We are not inspired enough to make a change. Guilt makes us feel even worse. Enter midnight binges. Doubt leads to defeat.

> *Whose end is destruction, whose god is the belly, and whose glory is in their shame, who think about earthly things.*
>
> *—Philippians 3:19 (WEB)*

Why do you have invalid thinking? Invalid thinking is based on doubt. It started in the Garden of Eden. Eve was deceived by Satan into thinking God did not have her best interests at heart. Doubt fueled her decision to take a bite of the apple, proving she did not trust God to meet all of her needs. Satan told her God was holding back on her. We are not very different in our thinking. Doubt fuels many of our food and exercise choices as well. Instead of recognizing we are slaves to our appetites, we are afraid of missing out on the next best thing. Yet, in our hedonistic selfie or I-dominated culture, we have no idea how to actually take care of our needs! Instead, we pursue our next fix with an entitlement mentality. We create problems in our minds we didn't even know we had, which is exactly what happened to Eve! We think we are treating ourselves, but in many cases we are just facilitating a slow death. Not only do we not know how to best love others, we don't even know how to love ourselves. In our race to put ourselves first, we have come in dead last. So how do we break free? How do we fix this invalid thinking?

> *Jesus said to him, "You shall love the Lord your God with all your heart, with all your soul, and with all your mind."*
>
> *—Matthew 22:37 (WEB)*

This is the commandment Jesus said was the most important. He is quoting Deuteronomy 6:5 where the word "might" was used instead of "mind." Loving the Lord with all of your might does not leave any room for doubt, which is a form of fear.

> *There is no fear in love; but perfect love casts out fear.*
>
> *—1 John 4:18 (WEB)*

Could you overcome your invalid thinking (doubts) by loving the Lord with all of your might? Could this teach you how to reclaim your energy in order to live victoriously? Could this teach you how to love yourself? Could loving the Lord your God with all of your might change your life? Could it set you free? The answer to all of the above is yes.

There is a reason Jesus cites the greatest commandment as "Love the Lord your God with all your heart, soul, and mind" instead of "Love the Lord your God as an ATM machine". Loving the Lord gets your mind off earthly things so you can attain eternal victory instead of suffering daily defeat. When we focus on earthly things, we are not free.

> *But I say, walk by the Spirit, and you won't fulfill the lust of the flesh.*
>
> *—Galatians 5:16 (WEB)*

Without faith, it's easy to get caught up in the "lust of the flesh." When you are lonely, discouraged, or stressed, you fill up on invalid things like junk food. Instead, if you have faith and "walk by the Spirit," you might join a church group to combat loneliness, read God's Word when discouraged, eat real food when you are hungry, and exercise when you are stressed. Stepping out in faith, instead of drowning in doubt, is what sets you free.

All You Need Is Love

You shall love your neighbor as yourself.
                                    —*Matthew 22:39 (WEB)*

This is the second part of the answer Jesus gave when He was asked what the most important commandment was. We are never going to love ourselves or others the way God intended unless we learn how to love God first. Loving your neighbor is second only to loving God. Your neighbor (friend, child, spouse) is not going to receive God's authentic love through you if you don't take the time to love God first. When you are told to love your neighbor as yourself, this assumes you love yourself! If you are a slave to your appetite, you are not loving yourself.

Many people go through life not knowing how to love because they have never experienced it. This type of love comes from a personal relationship with the Lord Jesus Christ. You may catch glimpses of it through others, but that's it. When you put God first, you are able to love others the way God intended. Only then can you love the most difficult people in your life, including yourself, as you are set free.

He Has a Reason to Be Jealous

"As I live," says the Lord, "to me every knee will bow. Every tongue will confess to God."
                                    —*Romans 14:11 (WEB)*

You serve a jealous God who will not tolerate second place. Many get so caught up with everyone else they do not even place God in their top five! Putting God first is not a suggestion but a command. It allows God's unlimited love to flow through you to others so you do not shortchange yourself or your loved ones. Many people literally knock themselves out trying to love their neighbor first but are limited in their human frailty. In this case, you can take one of two paths. You can become a loner because loving others is too exhausting and messy, or you can go the other extreme and forget to take care of yourself. Both paths lead to struggles with spiritual, emotional, and physical health, ultimately ending in defeat. Instead, the road to victory starts with loving God with all your heart, soul, and might. In order to be set free, you have to put more energy into seeking God and less energy into seeking everyone else's approval. To love God is to put Him in first place, treating Him as holy.

Because you didn't uphold my holiness among the children of Israel.
For you shall see the land from a distance; but you shall not go there.

—Deuteronomy 32:51–52 (WEB)

This was an admonition to Moses because he did not obey God and treat Him as holy. It cost him access to the Promised Land. One of the few times we treat God as holy is when we worship Him. Yet many avoid worship because they believe churches are filled with a bunch of hypocrites. This reminds me of an old joke: A pastor was outside of a new church, running around on a Sunday morning, trying to get the people outside of the church to come inside. He eventually got the attention of one couple, who finally said, "I am sorry, Pastor, but we are not going in there. We just don't want to be associated with a bunch of hypocrites." Without skipping a beat, the pastor said, "No problem! We have room for two more!"

He is still holy.

God saved you by his grace when you believed. And you can't take credit for this; it is a gift from God.

—Ephesians 2:8 (NLT)

First Things First

But seek first God's Kingdom, and his righteousness; and all these
things will be given to you as well.

—*Matthew 6:33 (WEB)*

Seeking God first helps you reclaim the energy you need to break free. If finding time to put God first seems overwhelming, realize this is the exact reason you need to put God first. You need to reclaim your energy. He will take care of the other things. I used to glance at the Bible as if I were reading the horoscope or cracking open a fortune cookie. I didn't get serious about seeking God until I realized I was not producing fruit. Efforts in many areas of my life were thwarted. I finally broke down and committed to seeking Him by spending a few minutes every morning reading the Bible.

I am the vine. You are the branches. He who remains in me, and I
in him, the same bears much fruit, for apart from me you can do
nothing.

—*John 15:5 (WEB)*

Reading the Bible first thing is like reading an owner's manual before pushing all of the buttons. If you do it first thing, it will be done before all of your buttons are pushed, thus giving you the right tools to better handle your day. It is the most effective time management tool you can employ. More importantly, it will set you free! Free indeed!

If therefore the Son makes you free, you will be free indeed.

—*John 8:36 (WEB)*

I started by reading only a few minutes a day. Now daily Bible reading has become the highlight of my day! Reading the Bible from front to back over a one-year period, instead of a passage or a quote here and there, is like the difference between being married to someone versus following them on Twitter. If you are feeling overwhelmed, rather than abandon ship, let's take baby steps. My passion for the Bible did not happen overnight either.

Is there an app for that? Well, of course there is. One of my favorite apps that I recommend to my classes is called First 5. It explains and applies the Bible in five-minute segments, and you can set it to your morning alarm. Several Bible apps with audible versions allow you to listen on your phone while working out, driving, or doing chores. An audible version coupled with reading is what finally got me over the hump, allowing me to start from the beginning. Just find five minutes and start somewhere. Reading the Bible fuels an excitement that only comes from the Lord. You can't buy it, and no one is selling it. Getting excited about today creates energy. Many people who are not excited about the Lord are not excited about anything.

"This girl runs on coffee and Jesus" is a shirt I wear when I do 5Ks, but it should really read, "This girl runs on Jesus and coffee." Waiting eagerly for what comes out of the "mouth of God" is what gets me out of bed each morning. I can't wait to open my Bible and breathe in the breath of Life. He is also speaking to you about your life. Are you listening?

> He wakens morning by morning, he wakens my ear to hear as those who are taught.
>
> —Isaiah 50:4 (WEB)

Once you surrender to Jesus, you are released from all other bondage. You just may not know it yet. There are many things in life we are not in control of, but you are free to decide whether or not to put God first, as well as what to put in your mouth. Inanimate objects have no control over you, including food. God gave humanity dominion over all things on this earth. It's not the other way around. Even the perceptions of reward or penalty your brain associates with a certain food or substance are ultimately up to you. If you view unhealthy foods as a reward, you will want them. If you view them as something that sucks the life right out of you, it will be easier to walk away. Believe me, after seeing the suffering my clients have been through, it is easier for me to walk away from a cupcake. Maybe you want to view excess sugar unfavorably but can't, at least not yet. In that case, ask God to show you the truth.

Pleasure versus Purpose

The thief only comes to steal, kill, and destroy. I came that they may
have life, and may have it abundantly.

—John 10:10 (WEB)

If you continually seek pleasure over purpose, you risk missing out on your
God-given potential. You will also remain a slave to your appetite. This is the
reason the numbers on the scale keep going up and up for us as a nation. All
these things we think we deserve (pleasure) are actually robbing us of our true
treasure (our purpose), keeping us enslaved. The next time you are tempted
by something derailing you from fulfilling your purpose, do what Jesus did
when He was tempted by the devil in the desert. He quoted scripture. If
Jesus quoted scripture to deal with temptation, I doubt you or I could come
up with anything better. The unsettling thing about Jesus's time in the desert
was that He was not the only one quoting scripture. The devil, who is a
fallen archangel, is also a biblical expert. He knows how to use, confuse, and
cause subterfuge with the Word of God. This is why you need to know God's
Word, so you can recognize deception. When Satan told Jesus to worship
Him, Jesus replied:

> *"Get behind me Satan! For it is written, You shall worship the Lord*
> *your God, and you shall serve him only." Then the devil left him, and*
> *behold, angels came and served him.*
>
> *—Matthew 4:10–11 (WEB)*

Jesus set the example of how to deal with the devil. He also reminded us to
"worship the Lord your God" and "serve him only." Instead of remaining
enslaved, quoting scripture will allow you to break free in order to fulfill your
God-given purpose for His glory. You don't even have to come up with a way
to say no. God has already done it for you.

FILLED OR FULFILLED?

Come to me, all you who labor and are heavily burdened, and I will give you rest, Take my yoke upon you, and learn from me, for I am gentle and humble in heart; and you will find rest for your souls. For my yoke is easy, and my burden is light.

—*Matthew 11:28-30 (WEB)*

God is not asking us to do more by spending time with Him. The devil wants you to think God is trying to overwhelm you with unrealistic demands. Instead, if we let God prioritize our days, we actually make an impact instead of just spinning our wheels. We also get to rest in the assurance that He is in charge, not us. We are set free. However, if we keep chasing the approval of others by saying yes to everything, we not only lose sight of what God's plan is for us, we waste a lot of time in bondage. I often hear how people don't have time to eat healthy and exercise because they are overscheduled. We want to believe we are doing all of the right things for all of the right reasons, but often we are really just seeking approval. When you seek God, you love others in the way God intended, whether you get their approval or not. This allows you to live a fulfilled life instead of just filling up your schedule with distractions. Asking the Lord to prioritize your life frees up energy you did not know you had, allowing you to make time for the things that matter. Chasing after other's approval enslaves you. Chasing after God sets you free!

WHY CAN'T IT BE YOU?

New clients ask, "Really, do you think I can actually lose the weight, get healthy, reach my goal, and get off of my meds? Do you think I can be healed?" They have struggled with weight issues their entire lives, or they have an injury or a disease. Unless there is some particular medical issue preventing them from improving when they actually eat healthy and regularly do some form of exercise, then the answer is yes.

The most important question to ask yourself is: "Do you want to be healed?" Think back to a time when you really wanted to strive for a professional or personal goal. How easy was it to talk you out of it? You can accomplish a lot within your own might and God's will. Imagine what you can accomplish within God's might and your will. Instead of choosing to do things within your own might, choose to love the Lord your God with all your might. See what His might can overcome in your life for His glory.

Repeatedly, my clients, who had the worst odds stacked against them, emerged with the biggest improvements. This made no sense until I realized that cancer, autoimmune disease, injury, depression, surgery, abuse, bankruptcy, diabetes, and even fat genes were no match for the Almighty. Whether these clients had started new careers, faced significant financial hardships, or gone through a recent divorce, they still lost weight. Neither did addiction, menopause, car accidents, or multiple surgeries stop them from losing weight. Even the busyness of raising special-needs kids, traveling for work, and serving in executive-level positions with frequent client dinners did not stop them from achieving their weight-loss goals. They all reclaimed their energy for God's glory, allowing them to fully serve His kingdom. He can help you do the same. God answers prayers.

> *This is the boldness which we have toward him, that, if we ask anything according to his will, he listens to us. And if we know that he listens to us, whatever we ask, we know that we have the petitions which we have asked of him.*
>
> *—1 John 5:14–15 (WEB)*

If you have struggled with emotional eating, sugar addictions, abuse, or a lack of motivation, you are not alone. There is no need to wait until your situation is ideal to start your weight-loss journey. The odds are stacked in your favor when you follow Christ, not when you have a problem-free life. Freedom is in Christ alone, not your circumstances.

> *Unless the LORD builds the house, the builders labor in vain.*
>
> *—Psalm 127:1 (NIV)*

Most people don't lose or maintain weight loss because they are in it for the wrong reasons. Your chance of success will be much higher if you recognize the problem and ask to be set free. Commit to asking for the strength to make healthier choices in order to reclaim your energy to serve the kingdom. If you are committed only to a number on the scale, you might give up after one week because you are a slave to the scale. If you stick it out longer and tweak certain areas, you can change your life. You will never know what you can achieve unless you commit. More importantly, with each new day, you can reclaim more energy. You can be set free.

MISPLACED MOTIVATION

> *How foolish can you be? After starting your new lives in the Spirit, why are you now trying to become perfect by your own human effort?*
>
> —*Galatians 3:3 (NLT)*

Many clients tell me all kinds of stories of deprivation, starvation diets, shots, fasts, boot camps, and extreme training sessions. I call these efforts misplaced motivation. This is a different kind of enslavement. Tremendous effort is put into things that are either not healthy or sustainable. It's great that a boot camp class allowed you to eat whatever you wanted in your thirties, but in your forties and fifties, you may not be able to exercise the pounds away. As the old saying goes, "You can't out-exercise a bad diet." As a matter of fact, I am seeing the truth of this statement in a new generation. The common theme among women in their twenties is to push their bodies too hard, either rebounding from deprivation diets or overeating and then overdoing it, winding up with an injury. You can learn how to avoid these pitfalls. If you are looking where to place your effort, this is where free will comes into play. You are as dependent on God when it comes to making healthier lifestyle choices as you are in making all other choices in your walk with Christ.

> *For bodily exercise has some value, but godliness has value in all things, having the promise of the life which is now, and of that which is to come.*
>
> —*1 Timothy 4:8 (WEB)*

Who's in Charge Here?

Indeed, we put bits into the horses' mouths so that they may obey us,
and we guide their whole body.

—James 3:3 (WEB)

You can control a horse's body by controlling its mouth, and there is not much the horse can do about it. You also are in control of your body when you control your mouth. You can control what you put in your mouth as well as what comes out of it. My biblical editor, Hailee Willhite, comments: "I know if I've eaten junk, I feel bad and become irritable and maybe not as nice. You speak what you eat." Mood and energy levels are affected by what you eat, which in turn affects your thoughts and beliefs. Negative thinking triggers inflammation in the body. Bad food not only triggers inflammation in your body, it also affects your mood, which then triggers more inflammation! Discouragement will leave you feeling lousy because you have made less than optimal food choices. Add sugar to the mix, and you discover you are now also on a blood sugar roller-coaster ride! We are also finding out the foods we eat can turn on and off certain gene expressions. What does this mean? Just because Grandma suffered with x doesn't necessarily mean we are doomed to the same fate if we make different choices. There are a certain series of events we have the ability to set in motion, or not, just based on what we put in our mouth. The same goes for what comes out of it.

Who is in control of your mouth? In the US Navy, when someone takes control of a plane, ship, or submarine, the following words are used: "I have the con," meaning I have control and am in command. Then someone replies, "You have the con." There is no question of who is in charge. Give God the con when it comes to your mouth, what goes in it as well as what comes out. Putting God in control sets you free.

GRACE INSTEAD OF GUILT

So now there is no condemnation for those who belong to Christ Jesus.

—Romans 8:1 (NLT)

The main reason Jesus came to earth was to take away the guilt of believers and replace it with grace. I am not talking about feeling guilty because you have gained weight or plowed through a quart of ice cream last night, but rather the guilt that fueled overeating in the first place. Oftentimes, guilt is unconfessed sin. Guilt is a tool the devil uses to enslave you. If you confess the sin, grace sets you free. Turn your guilt over to God in exchange for His grace. Victims of abuse often feel guilty because they feel in some way they were responsible for someone else's sin. This is another lie from Satan, which is discussed in depth during week six: hope.

To this end the Son of God was revealed: that he might destroy the works of the devil.

—1 John 3:8 (WEB)

THE WILL TO SUCCEED

This book is not about you white-knuckling it in order to succeed. It is about using your free will to ask Him for the power to be set free. You only have to make one big choice every day, and that is to love the Lord your God first. It will make the other little choices a whole lot easier. Instead of hanging out by the side of the pool like the invalid, you are going to actively pursue your freedom while giving yourself grace in the process. Upcoming chapters will teach you how to do this. It will not be easy, but I promise you it will be easier than what the devil wants you to believe. His lies and their consequences are intended to keep you enslaved and ultimately destroy you. Freedom is not easy, but it is better than the alternative. Freedom leads to victory.

Prudence

A prudent man sees danger and takes refuge; but the simple pass on, and suffer for it.

—Proverbs 27:12 (WEB)

Charles Dickens's *A Christmas Carol* has a character known as the Ghost of Christmas Future, who reveals a foreboding message to Scrooge. He shows Scrooge what the end of his life will look like if he continues on his current path. Scrooge desperately wants to know if it's too late for him to avoid this fate, but this ghost ain't talking. Fortunately, Scrooge gets his answer when he wakes up the next morning to another chance. He bolts out of bed with a madman's sense of urgency, on Christmas Day, embracing the fact that it's not too late. Everything looks different even though nothing has changed.

> *Jesus replied, "Very truly I tell you, no one can see the kingdom of God unless they are born again."*
>
> *—John 3:3 (NIV)*

I don't know if Scrooge was born again, but I do know he had a change of heart on Christmas Eve. By Christmas morning, he saw things in a completely different light, boldly headed in a new direction.

Imagine what it would be like if you had a visit from the Ghost of Christmas Future concerning your health. A few pounds today, after one too many special occasions or pity parties, can lead to obesity and disease tomorrow. You might think of your family history and hope to avoid a similar fate. My goal is not to scare you but to make you aware of the fact that time is a finite resource. Scrooge was fortunate enough to wake up to a second chance. Since you woke up this morning, you have also been given a second chance. It's not too late, but your future is closer than you think. As a matter of fact, it is one day closer.

Which future is it going to be?

Prudence is asking yourself, "What is the most likely outcome of what I am about to do?" *before* you do it. With our nation's obesity epidemic spiraling out of control, we are either not asking ourselves this question or ignoring the answer. So which future is it going to be? Unless we have a change of heart, our current view is already bleak, as it picks up momentum, heading straight toward our demise.

Prepare for Impact. Brace! Brace! Brace!

What if I told you I see people settling into relationships that are robbing them of their self-esteem? Or maybe they have just settled. What if I told you this was happening in our society at younger and younger ages? What if these relationships were making moms, dads, and children doubt their self-worth while also stealing their joy? Sometimes these relationships were even making them miss out on doing the things they used to love to do, or have never done, because they have already given up. What if these relationships were also preventing them from enjoying new adventures? What if I told you that lost opportunity was the norm instead of the exception? What if I told you they thought it was always going to be this way? What if I told you they felt trapped? What if I told you these relationships were hurting not only them but also future generations? What if I told you these relationships were also robbing God of His glory? What if I told you that one of the people I was talking about, in one of these relationships, was you?

Would you stay?

For how long?

Until it killed you?

Sadly, this is many people's relationship with food. Unfortunately, this is not all that I see. I see a lot of people of all ages suffering from something within their control yet living in bondage in our free country. I see families not going for bike rides or walks even though they are free to do so. I see the little girl at the park who told me she never gets to come to the park because no one will take her. I see moms embarrassed to swim with their kids because they don't want to wear a swimsuit. I see people who have no time for healthy eating and exercise. Yet I see scores of restaurants, known for all things unhealthy and supersized, overflowing with lines of people waiting insane amounts of time, spilling out the door, only so they can go in and make things worse. I see kids at school playgrounds who are unable to go across the monkey bars or climb a rope. I see long waits to get into doctors' offices, catastrophic health care costs, limited mobility, amputations, and medical personnel in physical therapy with bad backs, because patients are getting heavier. I see the largest number of diabetics and pre-diabetics the US has ever known, starting with young children. I see cancer feeding on sugar. I see obese children beginning life with something that is preventable. I see dreams abandoned before they have even had a chance to be imagined. I see teenage girls with eating disorders. I see moms with the same eating disorders. I see people believing weight loss surgery is the only way out, not really digesting the possible health consequences. I see women addicted to plastic surgery. I see grandparents having to make the choice between buying food or buying meds. I see people cutting themselves and their lives short.

Folks, this is not a drill.

I have witnessed scores of women break down and sob in front of me as they describe wasted years of misery for themselves and their families due to excess weight and health issues. I recently had a phone conversation with someone who spends $1,000 a month on diabetes medication. You may think, *Well, that's not me. I only have ten pounds to lose,* or, *I have better insurance.* Maybe your blood sugar is just a little high, not $1,000 worth! Like all problems, these start out small and manageable, until they become something you no longer recognize. Believe me, this person did not start out paying $1,000 a month. The price has gone up in more ways than one.

Sin always starts out as something manageable. Satan suggests the illusion that you will have just one cookie, drink, pill, and so on. I am not saying a cookie or a drink is evil, but if this is your weakness, this is what is going to be used against you. Instead of longing for something as if you can't live without it, remind yourself you are one cookie, drink, or pill away from actually living. Just one. If you do not pick up the next one, you have won, and God gets the glory.

My Doctor Made Me Do It

As a former health care administrator, certified by the American College of Healthcare Executives (ACHE,) I had the pleasure of working with many talented health care professionals. The majority of these individuals are in their profession to help people. Instead of blaming the medical community for our health care woes, we need to recognize we are getting what we demanded. We are basically saying, "Give me a pill/shot so I can still have my cake and eat it too." No one wants to hear their doctor lecture them on healthy eating, nor do most people listen. Most doctors do not have the time and have only a cursory knowledge of nutrition. Many medical professionals are struggling themselves. Yet the ones who are in it for the right reasons encourage others to do the same. My seventy-one-year-old friend Lee Truax and his wife, who both worked for years in prison ministry, have a doctor who jokes with them saying, "I like when you come in because I don't make any money off of you; you're too healthy." I love the honesty of this statement. The point here is the goal should be to see your doctor for wellness visits, immunizations, hereditary issues, or a diagnosis, not as a dealer supplying meds.

Although I am not a diabetes educator, people are referred to me who have type 2 diabetes. By God's grace, I have helped people decrease their meds/insulin and improve their blood work when nothing else worked. My diabetic clients have taught me a great deal. I used to ask why there was not more help for diabetics until I finally realized no one stands to profit if diabetics are healed. Businesses realize unhealthy employees cost more money. However, there is big money to be made by other businesses in keeping you addicted to sugar/fake sugars/processed carbs and then selling you the meds so you can eat some more. Why stop there? Why not buy into the illusion that a candy bar is healthy by throwing in some protein and renaming it an energy bar while increasing your sugar addiction? Now you're talking! I often hear that diabetes is really not about sugar. It's true that it is linked to excess weight and inactivity. However, what causes this excess weight? It is not coming from eating too many vegetables! It would be wonderful to blame the food manufacturers and pharmaceutical companies for this mess, but businesses are only selling what you and I are buying. The crime is when our children are targeted. You and I are big kids, but our children are just getting bigger and not in the right direction. Before you panic, thinking I never want you to have dessert again, there is a treat on the FVW plan every day. No one is going cold turkey, but there are certain guidelines that will make life a lot easier for you. The goal is for you to control your amount of dessert instead of the amount of your dessert controlling you.

Prudence is asking yourself, "What is the most likely outcome of what I am about to do?" *before* you do it.

If you can't have just one of something, it's time to move on, at least for now.

Love the Lord Your God

PRAY FIRST

Prudence is praying first. Although Cain gave an offering to the Lord just like his brother Abel did, the Lord liked Abel's offering better. The reason Cain's offering did not please the Lord was because it was not the "first fruits." Abel gave the first and best of what he had to the Lord. Cain gave leftovers. When you pray, give the Lord the first fruits of your day in the morning, not what you have left over when you get around to it—unless you want God to answer your prayers when He gets around to it with what is left over after the other 7.5 billion people on the planet. The point is to prioritize your time according to what is most important to you. If food is your struggle, schedule this time before you put food in your mouth. Pray first.

> But he answered, "It is written, Man shall not live on bread alone,
> but by every word that proceeds out of the mouth of God."
>
> —Matthew 4:4 (WEB)

Instead of living in defeat, you have been anointed and appointed to live like royalty. The Bible says there is a crown in heaven waiting for believers who have fulfilled their calling. How many crowns? There are five: the imperishable crown, the crown of rejoicing, the crown of righteousness, the crown of glory, and the crown of life, all found in the New Testament. Each crown is an award based on a different circumstance. The crown of life, for example, is for enduring trials, while the crown of righteousness is for loving the Lord's appearing. God bestows different crowns because He wants to reward your triumph over trials. Trials are your road to sanctification. If you are living a life full of trials, it is not going unnoticed. Satan is also paying attention. At your weakest moment, Satan is ready to convince you, "It's just one Christmas cookie!" This is why you need to pray first.

And no wonder, for even Satan masquerades as an angel of light.

—2 Corinthians 11:14 (WEB)

So how do you tell the difference between something disguised as good for you versus what is actually good for you? Pray first. Then ask yourself, "What is the most likely outcome?" If you are starving and haven't had lunch, then one cookie can turn into half of the bag before you know it. On the other hand, if you have eaten according to the plan all day, and it is time for dessert, go for it. Have one and enjoy it with your herbal tea or decaf coffee. If it turns out you still have a hard time with one, then decide if you are better off with something else next time. The point is there will always be the temptation to eat more than one. Decide which type of dessert makes it easier for you to hold the line. Personally, I would rather have a dark chocolate truffle than a Christmas cookie because that is a more satisfying way for me to end my meal.

Diet alone is not going to solve our problem. Our old thinking is not going to get us to our new destination. When Henry Ford built the first mass-produced automobiles, he couldn't use old thinking either. "If I had asked people what they wanted, they would have said faster horses" (Henry Ford). As my clients hear me say repeatedly, if a diet was the answer, I would be freely handing out copies of the diet, thus saving me the hassle of teaching a class and writing a book. However, if I did this, you would still be missing out on the truth, which is going to be your new way of thinking. The truth sets you free.

Then you will know the truth, and the truth will set you free.

—John 8:32 (NIV)

Change Your Brain

A Diet Is Not Your Destiny

Although there are many diets, a diet is not your destiny. Nobody wants to follow a diet, but everyone wants to find her destiny. This can only come from God. I have never had a person tell me it was a diet that gave her a life-changing ah-ha moment. Yet your epiphany will empower you to let go of whatever is holding you back from fullness of life. It is freedom to pursue your why.

> *Lay aside every weight and the sin which so easily entangles us, and let us run with patience the race that is set before us.*
>
> —*Hebrews 12:1 (WEB)*

If you want to win this race, you need patience. You also need to stop wasting your days looking at everything and everybody else. There are no life coaches, diagnostic exams, personality profiles, or career counselors who know the "why" for which you have been created, nor can they free you up to pursue it. These are external resources that can guide you along the path, but these resources are man-made and fallible. Look to the Word of God first, and then apply what you have learned. Why try to find your destiny from something man-made when you have the ability to seek it from the one who made you?

On Vanity

> *Vanity of vanities, all is vanity.*
>
> —*Ecclesiastes 1:2 (WEB)*

Most people go on diets because of vanity. Vanity may be a motivator, but clearly it is not enough to turn the tide on our obesity epidemic. I actually think that vanity is one of the things keeping most people fat. We compare ourselves to others and then get so discouraged that we just quit. If we worried less about how we looked on the outside instead of on the inside, we would all be better off. The word *vanity* is unflattering enough, but the NIV Bible's version of the above scripture gives the true intent of what was originally spoken, replacing the word vanity with the word *meaningless*. King Solomon points out that all pursuits without God are meaningless, and vanity happens to be chief among them. The emphasis we put on vanity is a huge waste of time. Why? Because it bears no fruit; we have nothing to show for it. We could blame all of this wasted time on the fact we live in a youth-obsessed culture, but vanity is nothing new. Does this mean we have been wasting huge amounts of time on meaningless stuff from the beginning of time? We seem to be a lot more obsessed with our bathroom scale than the passing of time, which is one of the reasons so much time has been wasted. However, just like Scrooge, our future is closer than we think.

Speaking of time, I have a tiny replica of Prague's astronomical clock called the Orlaj. This animated work of art has Vanity as one of its four main figures. She is holding a mirror, admiring herself. Greed, Death, and Lust are the other three prominent figures represented. Taken to extremes, vanity can kill; enter anorexia, bulimia, pills, and shots along with complications from multiple plastic surgeries. If it doesn't destroy your body, it will destroy your spirit. What a way to steal God's glory.

Each time an hour passes on this clock, the skeleton, representing death, rings a bell. The other animated figures all shake their heads, signifying they are not quite ready to depart. Since this clock was installed in 1410, not much has changed. Advertising campaigns today still revolve around these same four concepts. The difference is we now seem to celebrate most of these vices instead of despise them. The skeleton in the clock, representing death, is a reminder not only that life is short but also that these vices can destroy whatever days you have left.

One reason I feel called to share the message of FAITH VS. WEIGHT is to get the emphasis of health and weight management away from vanity and on to something more meaningful, like energy to serve the kingdom, which is where it belongs. It is not healthy to obsess over the scale or your physical appearance. Obsession is never healthy. It is a distraction from the devil. It allows only a fraction of what you have left over to serve, because most of your bandwidth is tied up in trying to reach unhealthy or unattainable goals. Others never experience the best you have to offer. When will we get to meet the real you, the one meant to bear fruit lasting into eternity?

> *You didn't choose me, but I chose you, and appointed you, that you should go and bear fruit, and that your fruit should remain; that whatever you will ask of the Father in my name, he may give it to you.*
>
> —*John 15:16 (WEB)*

INSPIRATION VERSUS MOTIVATION

Prior to creating FAITH VS. WEIGHT, it did not take long to figure out as a trainer what worked and what didn't. It wasn't any one diet or exercise plan. It had nothing to do with how old someone was or what disability or abilities they had. It didn't even matter what genetic background they came from in terms of fat genes or how hard or easy their life was. It almost seemed like clients in easier situations seemed to be less driven (a mañana attitude will never get you there). It didn't matter if they were rich or on financial assistance from the YMCA. Whether formerly obese, athletic or not, married or single, it did not seem to matter. It didn't matter if the person was an executive with an intense travel schedule, a retiree, or a stay-at-home mom, or one who works outside of the home. Nor did it matter how many hours a week they worked or how many kids they had. I will never forget the abdominal muscles I saw on a mom who had eight kids. With her workouts, she could probably take down a navy seal. So what matters? They all had one essential key ingredient. They were inspired. The reasons may have been good, bad, or even ugly, but they were inspired. The difference between inspiration and motivation is inspiration is intrinsic (internal), and motivation is extrinsic (external).

Inspiration is a hard thing to pin down. Yet it is the key to the kingdom when it comes to successful weight management. You may long for it but are not quite sure what it is or how to get it. Most people spend their whole lives chasing after it, but never seem to find it. Since many confuse motivation with inspiration, you may think it is something you can buy. This is because someone is always willing to sell motivation. If you pay for people or things to motivate you, then you will lose the weight, right? Yes and no. How many devices, apps, online programs, diet books, trainers, or gyms do we need to prod us along? Yet our problem is getting worse. Although these tools can make a difference, motivation is based on external circumstances. Instead, inspiration either creates circumstances, even in the most hopeless of cases, or it makes things happen in spite of the circumstances. Although it is not for sale, it is freely available. This is not to say there is no place for motivation. As a navy officer, I was motivated to get through enlisted and officer training, but like all motivation, it was temporary. Almost twenty years later, I make healthy choices because I am inspired. No one is making me do it. Yet I go out of my way to seek opportunities for healthy food and exercise choices no matter what situation I am in. This is what I want for all of my clients. This book cannot give you inspiration, but it will point you in the right direction.

How do you get the right kind of inspiration? Not the kind that has an ax to grind with an ex-husband? Only God can inspire us for the right reasons. Since I have been born again and started getting serious about reading the Bible every morning, I have not had a single day where I have had to ask God to inspire me. If you seek Him, He will inspire you! You will never find the inspiration that was meant for you and only you, or what is blocking you from experiencing it by looking out. Once you are inspired, it is much easier to change whatever behaviors are blocking you along your particular path. In terms of behavior, ask God to reveal what needs to go as well as what should replace it. Ask for His strength daily; that means one day at a time. Then in order to be successful, you must apply the common sense God gives you instead of jumping on whatever the latest diet craze is. Inspiration without common sense is like a ship without a rudder.

Offense versus Defense

The goal of this program is to put you on the offense concerning your health and weight management instead of always playing defense. Playing offense instead of defense is common sense. As an athlete prepares for a race, you need to prepare also. This is the race of your life, and you must have a game plan. Just like you have a strategy for work, you need a strategy for your health. You will switch from the emotional drama of weight management to a more strategic-based approach. This approach allows you to reclaim your energy and meet your objective. Prudence is playing offense instead of defense.

Strategic versus Tactical

Prudence calls for a strategy. Your battle with weight is a strategic problem (big picture) that you keep trying to solve at the tactical (details) level. Your strategy should be your driving force. Tactics change, but your overall strategy usually stays consistent. The purpose of this book, and hopefully for your life, is for you to have more energy to serve the kingdom, but what does this look like in your world? Your strategic outlook is the personalized answer to that question. Answer honestly since your results and long-term success depend on it. Ask God to show you what He wants you to do with your life. Your inspiration involves two components: you and the Lord.

1) Inspiration: Why am I seeking this reward? (strategic outlook)

(What is my reason for wanting to walk away from the temptation that is right in front of me?)

Since we are here to magnify God's glory, we need to reclaim our energy. The reward we seek is energy. Now we have to answer why we want more energy. This is where it gets personal. Not getting specific with the "why" is the reason most people fail at their weight loss attempts. The reason why you want more energy has to be inspired by God, not your scale. It might look something like this:

I want to have more energy ...

> to live out God's call in my life

> to do a better job of spending quality time with my family

> to be an authentic wife, mom, daughter, employer, volunteer, and so on

> to serve as God's hands and feet, not the fake ideal this world is selling

> to make better choices so I can control my blood sugar, since my doctor told me I am pre-diabetic

> to be able to handle and better prioritize my work and my children's extracurricular activity schedule

> to be more active with my kids since they are starting to also develop weight issues (This is way worse for me than having these problems myself. I keep telling myself they will grow out of it, but I didn't.)

> to have a better future for myself and for my family

> to take better care of myself and get off of my meds

> to show my children not only is it possible for me to get to a healthy weight, but it is also possible for them

> to break this generational stronghold

There are lots of reasons why to want more energy!

2) Illumination: What plan do I have in place to claim this reward? (tactical plan)

(What is going to help me walk away from the temptation right in front me that robs my energy?)

This is the second reason most people fail when tempting situations arise. They do not have a plan, or if they do, it is unrealistic. Most buy into whatever the diet of the day happens to be. Instead, each week you will gain confidence as you refine your plan in the "Change Your Life" section.

3) Transformation: How do I make this work in my life with my crazy schedule?

If I were drafting a contract, this is where I would get you to sign on the dotted line. You need a companion on this journey. Remember to walk with the Lord. It took a lifetime to get here, so do not expect someone else's results, who has been eating healthy and exercising for years, to be the same as your results in the first week.

If you apply these principles over time, you will wake up one day to your long-term goals. As my husband likes to remind me, "This is a marathon, not a sprint." In the meantime, every single day, and before every meal, you can set the short-term and immediate gratification goal of more energy. Losing a large amount of weight may seem like a pipe dream, but having more energy after your next meal, instead of less, is a blunt reality. Take this journey one meal at a time. There will be a lot of false starts. Think of these as teachable moments. When my clients are cruising along and then overdo it, they feel discouraged. I tell them to leave the guilt trip at the door since we don't have time to waste. Then I ask them how they felt physically after they polished off the last crumb. I already know the answer, but they need to know the answer. There is no better teaching tool than regret. I congratulate them on learning something I could never teach them with words alone. Then I ask them to rehearse the same scenario with a better outcome. You might think this is already obvious, but is it? We need to train our brains for victory. We need to remember the pain of failure and then mentally replace it with victory. If you are already eating healthy and in your groove, overdoing it is a much different experience than overdoing it on a regular basis. If you are overdoing it every day, you will barely notice the difference. However, when you start succeeding and then fall off the wagon, it smarts. Use this pain to remind yourself it is not worth it, and then imagine your next victory. The good news is you are only one meal or one walk away from it.

THE ROAD MORE TRAVELED

Below are some examples of plans that don't work. They come from not taking the time to answer question number one or two successfully or blowing off number three. Does any of the below sound familiar? (Keep in mind, these are common approaches, yet not one of these things mentioned below answers *what* or *why* when it comes to your reward or how you are going to claim it by walking away from the temptations right in front of you.)

> "I signed up for an extreme diet and marathon training program to fit into a dress for my sister's wedding. It worked. I lost ten pounds, but I gained it all back."

> "Feeling like I needed to lose weight, I decided to suck it up and sign up for boot camp classes! Once I started, I realized I was actually a couch potato and no longer the high school star athlete. Unfortunately, this wasn't such a great idea because now I have to get an MRI done on my ankle."

> "I decided to train for a triathlon to lose the pregnancy weight but injured my knee and stopped working out altogether. I ran track in high school and thought I could handle it, but apparently I jumped in too quickly."

Maybe you were a cheerleader, a basketball player, or the fat kid who never participated in any sports (which was me). Maybe you can't stand that you let yourself go or don't remember a time when you were not on a diet. Maybe you kept trying different plans but eventually blamed injuries, work, travel, family, obligations, genetics, aging, and stress for a lack of success. Or maybe you just gave up or never bothered in the first place.

Look before You Leap

If you choose strategy first, your plan will take a long-term outlook rather than a fly-by-night view, resulting in an unsustainable flop. Maybe a walking club is a better place to start than marathon training. My top client, who was recovering from two broken legs, lost seventy pounds without running one step! She consistently ate healthy and did the exercises she could do. The only place she ran to was the mall to buy new clothes.

Although running is not necessary, if you want to run, by all means go for it. However, you have to walk before you can run. Before I was able to return to running after a broken leg at age forty-five, I had to learn how to walk again without a limp. Next I learned how to walk on uneven surfaces and to walk the distance I wanted to run. Finally, I had to fast walk the distance I was planning to run and walk/run until I could build up to a sustained jog and then work on increasing my speed. When I started signing up for 5K races, I came in last place but eventually began winning races in my age group and in categories a decade younger than mine. I run on 100 percent Jesus power and glorify God with every breath and step, but I walked with Him for a long time, one step at time, before I ran a single step. That was also powered by Jesus.

I can do all things through Christ, who strengthens me.
—*Philippians 4:13 (WEB)*

Prayer Energy Equals Kingdom Energy

As emotional as your answer to your strategic outlook may be, over the next several weeks I advise you to redirect your emotional energy into prayer energy instead. When you pray, ask for help with focusing your energy into your plan instead of wasting it on negative emotions. Your success on your plan will be based on taking one tiny step after another, until someday you look back and realize you have scaled a mountain. This is only a function of time. The beginning is always the hardest part. Once you develop new habits, you can tweak them and experiment with even further gains. It has to become a habit first in order to establish a platform for success. Not all habits are bad, as some can actually save your life. The habit of walking on a regular basis allows you to start somewhere. However, before you take your first step, your plan needs to start from the place in your heart that is hurting. Otherwise you are wasting your time. Your area of greatest pain is where you will also find your greatest weakness. This is terrific news because with the Lord your greatest weakness can become your greatest strength. All you have to do is ask.

He gives power to the weak. He increases the strength of him who has no might.

—Isaiah 40:29 (WEB)

Habitual Destiny

We know that all things work together for good for those who love God, to those who are called according to his purpose.

—Romans 8:28 (WEB)

Your habits eventually lead to your destiny. Since your brain is economical by nature, when it figures out a shortcut, it will take it. This is for your survival, but it also sets off a series of chain reactions. When you commit something to habit, it frees you up to do other things. When you wake up in the morning, you do not need to think about brushing your teeth, right? Did you know there are actually several steps involved? First you need a job, money, and a car to go to the store to select a brand of toothpaste and a toothbrush. The habit of brushing your teeth saves you from major health problems. If your brain was still working on the basics of brushing your teeth, you would be exhausted by day's end. We would never move on to the next thing. Instead, you do not need to think about a habit; you do it by *default*. Since you are going to form habits anyway, why not form good ones by putting into practice the suggestions in this book?

Because your brain is highly efficient, it wants to go on autopilot so it is free to experience new things. Each time you practice doing something new for the first time, you form a new neurological pathway, and every time after that you reinforce it. This works both ways. The more you do not do something, the easier it is not to do it.

If you are convinced you cannot teach *an old dog new tricks*, consider what happens when you get a promotion. You learn new habits. You don't quit in the first few days because you are not a pro at your new position! Within a few months, you can do your new job in your sleep, but you had to start somewhere. Think of your healthy new lifestyle as a promotion!

Again, take all of your emotional energy and focus into prayer energy, asking for help to form better habits. This will result in greater kingdom energy. You will be practicing your faith and healthy habits for the remainder of this book and hopefully for the rest of your life. Prudence is forming habits that "work together for good."

Eat for Energy

Again, prudence is asking yourself, "What is the most likely outcome of what I am about to do?" *before* you do it. Keeping in mind what you just learned about habits, ask yourself if you really want to reinforce the choice you are about to make, before you do it. Just like I can't go shopping at Nordstrom and max out the credit card every week if I want to remain married, I can't go to a pot luck or buffet and grab everything in sight at every "special occasion" and wonder why my dryer keeps shrinking my pants. Unfortunately, most people view overeating as a consequence-free activity. They do not realize they are reinforcing certain bad habits and gaining weight. Instead, you want to eat to live, not live to eat.

ALL OR NOTHING

I can't tell you how many dieters tell me they are "all or nothing" people. This is exactly why they are perpetually on a new diet. Humans are not built for all or nothing. Systems are always striving to seek equilibrium. This is the case for human systems as well, whether you believe it or not. Some take dieting or exercise to an extreme and try to cut out everything or overdo it. This does not work in either direction. Certain aspects of your body will compensate for other parts not performing up to par. In a temporary situation, this isn't a big deal. When this goes on long-term, "Houston, we have a problem!" Things get thrown out of whack, whether due to repetitive movement injuries, extreme diets, or sugar addictions resulting in chaos. Balance is the opposite of chaos. Peace sets the stage for balance just as balance supports peace. The nutrition plan I use with my clients balances out their blood sugar, helping them to create sustainable habits. Prudence is not an "all or nothing" mentality.

My goal for my clients is to keep their blood sugar in check since this is something that can easily be managed in most cases by creating good eating habits. If you keep your blood sugar under control by not overdoing sugar or carbs (even healthy ones), you will also lose weight. This is a two for one. But wait, there's more … you will also have sustained energy. I am not claiming this will cure anything. I am not a physician or a nutritionist. I am just a trainer who helps people lose weight.

The Lord has allowed me to participate in magnifying His glory using this plan to help others create more energy to serve His kingdom. The results are all quantifiably proven both in terms of weight loss and improved blood work when clients have their routine wellness visits. Besides losing weight, having their doctor's confirmation that the FVW plan is improving their numbers elates my clients. That's good enough for my clients, and it's good enough for me. I enjoy receiving their victory texts! However, since I am always in pursuit of helping my clients live healthier lives, I pay attention to breakthroughs in nutrition and exercise science. In pursuit of excellence, this plan may look slightly different in three years or next week, depending on the next scientific breakthrough, but the faith part remains the same.

Jesus Christ is the same yesterday, today, and forever.

—Hebrews 13:8 (WEB)

The characteristics of real food also stay the same. An apple is still an apple. Because God created real food for us to eat, this plan is based on real food. That is not going to change either. However, all bets are off with our processed food supply. The standard American diet (SAD) is like playing Russian roulette.

THE HALO EFFECT

The halo effect, when applied to food products, is when we assume an entire product is healthy because one or two healthy ingredients have been added. I call these food products pseudo-healthy. In my opinion, pseudo-healthy foods are public enemy number one! Why bother eating real food when you can just buy a shake or a bar advertising omega-3 and fiber that tastes like a chocolate chip cookie? Fake healthy foods are one of the fastest-growing markets in the food industry. Over the years, I have been approached to sell some of these items to "enhance" my clients' results, but I have refused. I believe God made the perfect food for our bodies. Do we really think we can do better? We can measure only the things we know how to measure. Do we really know the long-term health effects of any of these fake foods?

Do you want to live to one hundred, or are you just trying to get through today? Most centenarians were raised on real food. It doesn't take a rocket scientist to figure this one out since we did not market fake foods until the 1970s. Populations living longer in parts of the world other than the United States mostly stick to traditional (real food) diets. With all the money we spend on health care, you would think the US would be leading the charge toward better nutrition, but we are not.

Many processed foods may have one or more nutrients listed or added to improve the product's overall nutritional value. However, in most cases, the rest of the product is loaded with unhealthy ingredients, including real or fake sugars. Even if a product has good ingredients like fruit, the sugar content is through the roof because it contains fruit juice, which is fruit minus the fiber, or real fruit but often not in the amount nature intended. Fake sugars can be even worse than real sugar because you really do not know the long-term effect the fake sugars will have on your health or your ability to control sugar cravings. Although you may feel less hungry temporarily, it may spur other cravings or cause other problems, sabotaging your health. Just because something claims to help with weight control does not mean it is automatically a waist-friendly food.

The halo effect can also apply to real food. Although dry roasted nuts are healthy for your heart and may have no added sugar, they are still high in fat. Because you can easily lose track while eating, why not buy hundred-calorie bags of nuts or make your own? Read nutrition labels to figure out what a hundred calories of any nut looks like. (Without shells, one hundred calories is about two tablespoons.) I usually get pistachios with the shells on since this slows me down. Grains are another food category that can easily be overeaten. Just because brown rice and oatmeal are real whole foods doesn't mean they will not negatively affect your blood sugar, causing you to crave more carbs or sugar, depending 100 percent on the timing and the amount.

I learned this the hard way after many years of trial and error. However, it turned out to be a real breakthrough for this diet. You will learn all about suggested complex carbohydrate timing and amounts.

The halo effect also applies to health food stores. Repeatedly, my clients share that they subconsciously believe things sold at health food stores generally have healthier ingredients so they do not have to worry as much about portion sizes. In most cases, the ingredients are much better than the processed stuff, but a cupcake is still a cupcake. Cut the cupcake in half for a dessert after dinner but realize it is still a cupcake. Something does not qualify as a "health" food based solely on the fact it was purchased at a health food store. Prudence is deciding on the timing and amount before putting sugar on your plate.

You Can Have Whatever You Want!

"All things are lawful for me," but not all things are profitable. "All things are lawful for me," but not all things build up.

—*1 Corinthians 10:23 (WEB)*

One of the main points I emphasize with my clients is that they can eat whatever they want, as much as they want, for as long as they want, if that is what they *really* want. I then have them visualize an all-you-can-eat stand on an ocean boardwalk. It looks exactly like the ones where you buy funnel cakes. The aroma is wafting through the ocean air. Can you smell it? I tell them that all of the items are free, and their favorite decadent foods are all there and will never run out. I then ask them to picture themselves in front of it, sitting with their family eating as much as they want, at their current weight.

We then fast-forward to another option of them alongside the same ocean-front with their family listening to seagulls and breathing in the tropical air on a sunny day. Can you smell it? Except this time they are not sitting; they are all racing toward the ocean, running right past the funnel cake stand. This time, they can't wait to jump in the ocean! They have been eating healthy and exercising regularly for the past year, bursting with reclaimed energy. Their children are so excited they are joining them for some fun in the sun because, for the first time, their parents are at peace with their bodies.

Now tell me, which option do you *really* want?

I think you can guess which of the scenarios my clients select. The first point here is that what you think you want in the moment is not what you really want as your destiny. The second point is that no one else is in control of your eating habits. No one has the power to make you eat or not eat. You can't even blame this one on the devil. Do you blame a diet, trainer, or somebody else as the reason you can't have a certain food? This mentality is what is keeping you fat. It is time to stop blaming others for why you are making certain choices. Making better choices is not a penance because it leads to a reward. Own it. This is why identifying with your reward is so important. It's your choice and nobody else's. Do you want to be healed or not?

What better place to go for inspiration to exercise than a Sylvester Stallone movie? There is a scene from the 2015 movie *Creed* where Rocky Balboa gestures toward a mirror that Adonis Creed (the illegitimate son of his former opponent, Apollo Creed) is focused on while shadowboxing. **Rocky tells Creed,** "You see this guy here? That's the toughest opponent you're ever going to have to face. I believe that's true in the ring, and I think that's true in life." Well said, Rocky! The visual impact of this statement is so powerful because Adonis Creed is literally shadowboxing himself, looking himself straight in the eye in the mirror. As Christians, we often say Satan is our toughest opponent, but this is only half of the story. There is no reason to give him more credit than he deserves. Because when Satan shows up with his lies, you are the one who ultimately chooses whether or not to believe them or fight back.

So I run with purpose in every step. I am not just shadowboxing.

—*1 Corinthians 9:26 (NLT)*

Jesus was not only resisting temptation for Himself in the wilderness, He was protecting his Father's honor by not allowing God to be robbed of His glory.

His Father's glory was more important to Him than His own life. Clearly, we see this on the cross. Satan's primary objective is to rob God of His glory. You just happen to be in the crosshairs, as are all followers of Christ. God is being robbed of His glory when His children believe the lies of Satan over His truth. If you want to believe you have no options or you will never be able to make healthy choices on a regular basis, you are denying the Father His glory. The victor has already claimed the victory. Your job is to remind everyone, including yourself, of this fact for His glory. You are not here to blame but to reclaim.

Temptations versus Cravings

The plan I share with you helps you manage your blood sugar, allowing you to no longer be a victim to sugar cravings. You will still be tempted, but you will no longer crave sugar. There is a huge difference. For this to happen, you have to follow the plan. View this as a three-day science project. Three days usually gives you enough time to feel a difference. It is also a manageable time period. Although everything in this plan occurs in a specified amount at a certain time of day, including dessert, the plan is super simple. Remember to follow portion sizes in order to keep your blood sugar in check. By controlling your blood sugar, you will be able to control your cravings from a physiological standpoint. If you justify that you will have just a little sugar here and there in addition to the times specified on this plan, you will only be shadowboxing yourself. You can liken this to a smoker who is trying to quit but decides to have one cigarette here and there at random times. It is torturous to do either sporadically. Clients tell me it is easier to exercise on a regular basis. Why? The same reason you would not want to start a brand-new job every week. Things become easier once they become a habit. This keeps your body from having to repeatedly start all over again. Prudence is following the plan.

CRAVINGS

I view cravings as physiological, while temptations are psychological. We are physically drawn to them. If you continually eat sugar, fake sugars, and carbs, you will crave them all day. Your body will always be looking for the next fix. It is so easy to eat sugar and excess carbs in their various forms even if you think you are a healthy eater. Before you even walk out your front door, you may already be on a sugar/carb high because most products have excessive sugar/carbs in them. Are you making "healthy" smoothies loaded with fruit sugars containing as much sugar as a can of soda? When you eat and drink sugar all of the time, you will crave it all of the time. This is not all in your head. Studies show how your brain lights up like a Christmas tree when you ingest sugar. It makes it difficult to eat a healthy salad (one not loaded with more sugar) for lunch if you had a Danish at 10:00 a.m., or even after a "healthy" bar promising to give you all-day energy. The earlier in the day you start eating sugar, processed foods, and certain carbs, the more likely you are to crave them all day. Then you wind up beating yourself up, wondering why you can't do better. Without realizing it, you may have eaten more than a couple of candy bars' worth of carbs in the form of sugar/carbs due to your "healthy" smoothie, cereal, bar, or coffee loaded with sweeteners. Reminder: sugar is a carbohydrate.

Fake sugars, even the ones labeled "natural," are often worse than real sugars when it comes to perpetuating cravings. The jury is still out as to what their long-term effects are on your body. After eating this "healthy" (that's what it says on the box) item, you most likely will crave more sugary foods later. Even the fake sugars claiming not to affect insulin levels keep the taste of something sweet in your mouth, leading to more cravings. A breakfast with added sugar / fake sugars does the same thing. This is the reason many say eating breakfast makes them hungrier. Eating protein along with the right amount and type of carbohydrates and fat will satisfy you in the morning instead of leaving you starving one hour later.

You may think skipping breakfast equals less calories, but this often leads to afternoon or evening binges. I never skip breakfast. I may not eat it first thing, but I have it as early as I can. If you feel hungrier a few hours later after eating a balanced breakfast, this is because your metabolism is turned on. This is a different type of hunger than the one experienced coming off of a sugar high. When you fail to start your day with a healthy breakfast or jump-start your morning with a sugar roller-coaster ride, you set yourself up for failure the rest of the day. If the sugar highs were worth it, you would be running around spreading joy all day instead of your waistline. Many obese people skip breakfast.

Don't fall into the trap of grabbing pseudo-healthy sugary bars or drinks, jump-starting a sugar roller-coaster ride before the day even gets started, or take the "high road" and skip breakfast all together ("But I'm not hungry when I wake up …"). The reason so many people do not have an appetite for breakfast is because they are eating junk late at night. Then they skip breakfast and go to work. Lo and behold, the office break room or teacher's lounge never seems to disappoint. Everyone eventually gets hungry for breakfast. If they didn't, there wouldn't be a doughnut shop on almost every corner of every strip mall. Of course, there is always a well-meaning coworker or friend who adds to your temptation by buying extra doughnuts to share. Somebody is eating all of these doughnuts, even though no one is hungry for breakfast. You might be first in line for doughnuts if you do not eat a satisfying breakfast. If doughnuts are your favorite food on the planet, no problem. We have a category for them on this plan. It is called dessert, because that is what they are. One half a doughnut for dessert is plenty.

Since you eventually get hungry for breakfast, you need a plan. On the days you can't eat breakfast right away, I have suggestions for an energizing two-ingredient hot cacao drink in the appendix that will keep hunger at bay until you can eat. I also have a pre-workout drink suggestion for the days you work out in the morning. I recommend you eat breakfast right after your work out or at least before you are around mass temptations. This means have it ready for after your workout or before the office boardroom doughnut meeting. There are plenty of grab-and-go options listed.

Temptations

Temptations are psychological. Once you are no longer inundated with sugar all day and have been following this plan, you will notice the difference between a temptation and a craving. My clients tell me when they come across foods they used to crave before this program, they may be tempted but no longer automatically grab it without thinking. They are able to walk away. When you are tempted, you should realize that what you eat at this meal will also affect what you crave for your next. That makes it easier to walk away since most people want to avoid the sugar roller coaster they have finally gotten off of. However, if it is something you want to have as a dessert, just wait for dessert and have it in the appropriate amount. Having dessert after a FAITH VS. WEIGHT dinner in a small amount is part of your plan. This is usually enough to get over it.

> *No temptation has taken you except what is common to man. God is faithful, who will not allow you to be tempted above what you are able, but will with the temptation also make the way of escape, that you may be able to endure it.*
>
> *—1 Corinthians 10:13 (WEB)*

When I am tempted, I think about how I am going to feel after I eat whatever is tempting me. This has become a habit. In other words, I automatically ask myself, "What is the most likely outcome?" before I do it. Since I really don't have time to squander my energy, this works for me. I also may hit the play button on a Bible verse I have in my head, and I tell my clients to do the same. The Bible verse I have memorized is tied to my strategic outlook and reminds me to stay on track. Again, this is why your strategic outlook is so important. It has become automatic for me and many of my clients, and it will become automatic for you also. In my case, my dreams, otherwise known as my "why," are way too big to have inanimate objects suck the life out of them or me. There is a lot of work to do, and I need all of the energy I can to do it! Now that tempting thing really does not look so tempting after all once I am reminded of my reward to have more energy to serve the kingdom!

Commit your actions to the LORD, and your plans will succeed.

—Proverbs 16:3 (NLT)

Finding something you are more excited about than food is a great place to start. Getting specific as to why you want more energy to serve the kingdom based on what God is calling you to do is why you define your reward in the first place. Commit to the Lord and see what kinds of plans and doors He opens for you when you rededicate the body He gave you to serve as His hands and feet (the reason we have a body in the first place).

Maria's Bible Verse:

"You have been faithful with a few things; I will put you in charge of many things. Come and share your master's happiness!"

—Matthew 25:23 (NIV)

When I am tempted, I repeat my Bible verse, which is based on my strategic outlook.

Maria's Strategic Outlook:

I want more energy to:

> love the Lord my God with all my heart, soul, and might

> love my neighbor as myself, starting with my family, church, greater community, and wherever else I am called in this world

> share the Good News

> serve with a cheerful and grateful heart

> start a *glory movement* (I want to see Christians reclaim their energy in order to serve the kingdom for His glory. I want you to be one of them!)

I am an older mom with younger kids married to a husband who is almost four years younger than me. I am the oldest in my house. I can't afford to be in a food coma. I can't afford anything that robs my energy. Loving the Lord my God and my family makes me want to make healthy choices so I have the energy to serve Him and them. As mentioned, I began my early years overweight, but by God's grace, I have been delivered, and I don't plan to end up there. I have a family history of obesity, diabetes, cancer, and heart disease, but I am hoping to live as fully and disease-free as long as the Lord permits. I plan to make the best choices for as long as I can. I have seen the detrimental effects of not taking care of health, both in my own family and from working in hospitals, and I don't want to settle. I want to enjoy the time with my family today and cherish being a grandmother tomorrow. I want to have the energy to interact with my grandchildren, go on international mission trips, do a sprint triathlon, continue to compete in 5Ks, swim, bike, walk/jog, and share the message of FAITH VS. WEIGHT for as long as the Lord allows. I want to spread the Gospel by sharing it and living it. I want to share my passion of living a healthy lifestyle. I am excited about getting you excited about your health, which is fulfilling my calling and helping you to fulfill yours for His glory!

Why do you want more energy?

(Hint: I didn't know any of this until I spent time in His Word. If you don't know your answer, put this book down and start reading the Bible). Choose your strategic outlook.

THE PROMISED LAND

"You have lived long enough at this mountain."

—Deuteronomy 1:6 (WEB)

One estimation suggests the trip to the Promised Land was only an eleven-day journey, but because of a lack of faith, it wound up taking the Israelites forty years. When it comes to diets, it's easy to feel as if we are going around in circles for years as well. We find staunch low-carb advocates, Ketogenic diet fans, vegans, raw foodies, and even bariatric surgery. We also find packaged food delivery companies, HCG shots, and pills. Then before we know it, we find we are running out of money! I have had clients who have tried all of these methods, and you may have tried one of these yourself. When I look back and ask, "What is the perfect diet?" I remember this old saying: there are three sides to every story: his side, her side, and the truth, which often lands somewhere in the middle.

When I first questioned what the perfect diet would be, I couldn't help thinking about centenarians. Surely they must eat a perfect diet. Well, not necessarily. On top of that, there is not one single diet centenarians follow. The Okinawan diet did not include Mediterranean dishes, just like the French centenarians are probably not slurping down Japanese miso soup. However, you can probably bet there are not many obese centenarians. As you examine cultures around the world and some of their centenarians (who supposedly have worse health care than we do), you will find they eat full fat, animal fat, whole grains, and even small amounts of processed carbohydrates and sugar. Some also have alcohol, while others do not. There is no one successful diet. However, they do have some things in common. Most are not on a diet, and eating seems to be a secondary instead of primary activity. They just eat a certain way that works for their bodies and not against them. They also typically have strong spiritual and social connections. Centenarians also tend to keep moving. Although most may not be running a marathon, they are not sitting all day either. The only real common theme of these lifestyles is balance. There is a certain rhythm of habits and rituals that have been reinforced over time. In other words, they are not eating like Americans. They are not overdoing it at the all-you-can-eat buffet, and they are not abusing alcohol or overeating sugar. Most centenarians are not restricting any food groups. So where does this leave you? What does God have to say about your diet?

THE PERFECT DIET

> *Jesus said to them, "My food is to do the will of him who sent me, and to accomplish his work."*
>
> —*John 4:34 (WEB)*

Before you take a bite of whatever this world has to offer, this is what you are to consume first. You are here to do His will and accomplish His work, not your own. This is also a reminder that you are completely dependent on Him for all sustenance in order to do His will and work. He provided manna in the wilderness to teach man to depend on Him alone since food is something man could not live without. You couldn't hoard manna either. There was no buying manna in bulk; it would rot. This was a one-day-at-a-time type of dependence on the Lord. Whether you realize it or not, you are in the same boat.

> It is written: "Man shall not live by bread alone, but by every word that proceeds out of the mouth of God."
>
> —Matthew 4:4 (WEB)

The FAITH VS. WEIGHT Diet

There is an old joke about exercise that also applies to diets.

Question: What is the best type of exercise?

Punch line: The one you will actually do!

The same thing applies to healthy diets. A healthy diet works only if you will actually follow it. Jesus met people where they were. However, He did not leave them there. When I first started out as a trainer, I wanted everyone to eat what I thought was the perfect diet. I was focused on egg white veggie omelets for breakfast. There is nothing wrong with omelets, except that some people don't like veggies in the morning, or eggs, or cooking, or breakfast, or mornings. That doesn't mean there aren't other healthy options. I also learned I had a crowd who loved smoothies. I fought this crowd for a long time until one day I decided to make blood-sugar-friendly smoothies, and this was another breakthrough. Eventually, the plan wound up being the easiest for most clients; they were able to follow it and happy to do so. In their own words, they told me they "craved" their smoothies and were shocked because they did not feel deprived when they went out for meals.

The reason they were not craving other foods was because they got a handle on their blood sugar.

Repeatedly, I went back to the drawing board and listened until there was compliance. I discovered what was reasonable in their life at every meal and snack so the expectations were not unrealistic. My number one job is to get my clients interested in taking care of themselves so they can have more energy to serve the kingdom. I cannot do this alone and pray for wisdom with each new client. Initially, change can be challenging. However, once clients start feeling better and seeing results, they start initiating further changes on their own.

When trying out a new diet, depending on the stage of change you are currently in, you may be ready to jump in, or you may have to start out by working on one meal a day. In this case, try focusing on the same meal for three days. Whether it's the daily doughnuts or pizza, keep the following in mind: if you show up starving, you will leave stuffed. To be successful, you never want to be in situations where there are temptations (which is practically everywhere) when you are starving. You are fighting evolutionary urges when you do this, setting yourself up for failure. If you want to win, help your body have a fighting chance by filling up on the good stuff so you are less vulnerable to the bad. It is actually easier to follow all of the plan rather than part of the plan. This may sound counterintuitive but it is not, because the main goal is to control blood sugar. If you "cheat," you are not only cheating on your current meal but setting yourself up to fail at the next one because you will be fighting the blood sugar roller coaster. Remember it is easier to try the whole plan for three days than to rip the Band-Aid off slowly. You can do anything for three days.

Primary goal: magnifying the glory of God by reclaiming your *energy* to serve the kingdom!

My Clients' Idea of the Perfect Diet

- delicious

- nutritious
- convenient
- flexible (you can do it while you are at restaurants, entertaining, or traveling)
- fast
- affordable
- easy
- allows favorite foods

My Idea of the Perfect Diet for My Clients

I want the same things listed above for my clients, with some elaboration:

- Proper hydration: hydration comes first, not last.

- Proper satiation: controlled blood sugar equals fewer cravings.

- Proper nutrition: well-nourished within the appropriate number of calories.

- Four to six meals a day: four is fine as long as you are getting enough of the right type of calories without binging or making bad choices.

- Lean protein: enjoyed at key times throughout the day for alertness and muscle recovery.

- Healthy plant-based fats: Specific amounts at specific times of day to beat sugar addiction. These fats are delicious and lead to satiation besides contributing to overall nutritional needs.

- Carbohydrates: Eat vegetables at the times of day you have easy access to them (lunch salad bar), and eat low glycemic fruits in order not to spike blood sugar. Eat higher-carb options later in the day. This allows you to burn fat during the day while maintaining high energy levels, as well as keep cravings in check.

- Sugar: Limit sugar intake by limiting the amount of processed sugar and carbs eaten all day by eating according to the plan. You will be satisfied with a smaller amount of sugar after dinner. Once you are no longer controlled by blood sugar swings, you can actually make a decision. When choosing an appropriate amount, you can control your dessert instead of your dessert controlling you!

In order to do this:

You have the option of enjoying starchy complex carbohydrates in the evening only. (This helps with sugar cravings and energy all day long while also improving sleep.)

You have the option to have sugar, but only at specific times of day: Pre-workout: add one tablespoon of honey to a pre-workout drink (see eating timing and tips chart). After dinner: enjoy a hundred-calorie portion-controlled dessert.

Broth-Based Soup

Broth-based soups help people feel fuller with fewer calories. A favorite is turkey bone broth, but any broth-based soup will suffice. Bone broth soups have more protein than other broth-based soups. Another soup with protein is miso soup. Miso has tofu, which is heralded as a health food by some and demonized by others. Do what works for you. Soups are a great start to a meal on a winter's night. Another good option is French onion soup. I usually order French onion soup without the bread. I would rather spend those calories sharing a small dessert at a French restaurant than eating the bread in the soup.

Dinnertime is the perfect time to have a favorite food not on the list. If we start straying early in the day, it will be harder to get back on track. Do not skip meals or snacks! You don't ever want to go into dinner starving. Having a favorite at dinner does not mean eating more food. It means substituting your favorite food under the proper category. At dinner, there are five categories: protein, fat, veggies, starchy carbs, and dessert. A small amount of cheese or fruit is optional. Don't forget to add flavor with garlic, onions, herbs, and spices to go from ordinary to extraordinary.

If starchy carbs are your thing, then substitute your favorite food item for the carb and dessert option. Since pizza is a starchy carb, what would this look like at a pizza place? A grilled chicken salad with olive oil would count as your protein, vegetable, and fat. A slice of pizza would count as your carb and dessert. Instead of pizza, you could also have a portion of lasagna, pasta, or quiche. If one of your favorite foods is in the protein category, an example might be substituting one piece of fried chicken for your protein option and skipping dessert. You would still have your vegetable, healthy fat, and starchy carb at dinner.

This is not a daily recipe for health but occasionally allows for an old-time favorite. The frequency is entirely up to you. Eat whatever you want as often as you want but just make sure it is really what you want! Remember the previous beach example. Since I would rather have dark chocolate for dessert, I have that instead of pizza, fried chicken, or quiche.

Cheese Please!

Many dieters eliminate cheese, getting so restrictive they wind up later overdoing it on pizza, cheesy dips, or an extra piece of cake, which are all more calories than just adding two tablespoons of cheese. Dressings claiming to be blue cheese have very little actual cheese in them. However, almost all have sugar. Use real cheese instead of dressings with the word cheese in them. Although some people have issues with dairy, they still seem to eat a lot of cheese. On the breakfast/snack and lunch/dinner plan, you will see small amounts of various cheeses available. If you use cheese as suggested on the charts, you are basically using it as a condiment instead of as a main course. Small amounts of high-quality cheeses allow for a wonderfully rich, decadent flavor while costing only a minimal number of calories. Go for cheeses with a sharp flavor, and you will need less.

I finally realized whenever I wanted a slice of pizza, I wasn't really craving pizza, I was craving melted cheese. Instead of eating pizza, I decided to melt two tablespoons of real shredded parmesan on broccoli or melt gorgonzola on a chicken breast. I also add one tablespoon of extra virgin olive oil as my plant-based fat. These combinations are delicious. Ask for cheese on the side at restaurants since many tend to overdo it. More is not better. This way, you can add two tablespoons yourself. If you order an omelet with melted cheese in it, eat only half of the omelet. Enjoy a few slices of avocado on the side.

The Mediterranean diet, which is highly rated, uses small amounts of cheese as a condiment. People are able to stick with it without feeling deprived. However, many people need more guidance than just generally following a diet that includes certain types of foods. They need to know how much and when. Besides cheese, the other dairy products worth mentioning are yogurt and cottage cheese. Yogurt and some cottage cheeses have probiotics, but the latter also has the added bonus of having a higher protein content. The breakfast/snack chart has ideas for both yogurt and cottage cheese in smoothies. If you decide instead to use yogurt or cottage cheese as a condiment, one fourth cup is approximately forty calories. Top off your omelet with one-fourth cup of Good Culture cottage cheese, which is grass fed and has probiotics. Use grass-fed Greek yogurt mixed with olive oil, lemon, and black garlic to make a creamy salad dressing. Black garlic is fermented and not as strong as white, with a more savory flavor.

Although people don't always think of it as dairy, butter also falls in this category. Try Kerry Gold Light. You can substitute one teaspoon instead of cheese and think of it as a condiment to drizzle over an entree. You can also use one teaspoon of ghee instead of cheese as a condiment. Don't forget to add a hundred calories of plant-based fats as shown on all charts. Milk has high sugar content and can cue sugar cravings all day if you have it in the morning. If you want milk, drink it at night. If you are not ready to give up milk in your morning coffee, try one tablespoon of coconut butter or one tablespoon of cream. Limit coconut oil. It has a higher saturated fat content than coconut butter without any additional taste benefit.

Your lack of perfection is why Jesus came! Trying to do everything perfectly often leaves us with nothing, because perfect is unattainable. You may then get discouraged and go downhill. This is true in all categories, and dieting is no exception. You may tend to last a few days on a diet or lose a ton of weight only to gain it all back because no one can maintain a super-restrictive lifestyle forever. This is another reason most diets fail. However, this plan is a little looser, on purpose! It is meant to be an attainable lifestyle. If you fall into the category of being a perfectionist or triple type A, do not be penny wise and pounds foolish with calories. Little splurges (that do not contain sugar) during the day can go a long way. Being calorie conscious, some may want to skip the fifty calories added by the additional two tablespoons (half ounce) of cheese crumbles. They do not realize this may save them from later faceplanting into eight hundred calories of nachos supreme. If cheese is not your thing, nuts are heart healthy and another great choice if used as a condiment on a salad, as long as they are not candied. One tablespoon of roasted or raw nuts is approximately fifty calories. Nuts or cheese in small amounts are both fine options.

You need to know which splurges will satisfy you and which will derail you. Whenever I hear "everything in moderation," I hear good intentions, but I also realize many people do not necessarily know what things they should consume in moderation. Sugar and starchy carbs earlier in the day make it harder to be moderate the rest of the day, so avoid little splurges that involve sugar and starchy carbs during the day. At night, you can incorporate them within the plan. It makes it much easier to control the amount when you are following this plan and not eating them all day. The same logic applies when having a hundred-calorie dessert every day. Popcorn or chocolate can be an after-dinner dessert as long as you keep close to a hundred calories. Just remember to keep it as a dessert, which means after dinner. If you have your hundred-calorie treat after a balanced FVW dinner instead of before it, you will have a much easier time stopping there. This is not about your willpower. This is about your blood sugar. This plan helps keep your blood sugar in check.

Replace Liquid Calories with Coffee or Tea

Replacing one drink a day with a healthy substitute is how we transition from sodas: diet or regular, energy drinks, or coffees that resemble ice-cream shakes. Trying to cut everything out at once can backfire. Coffee and tea are fine. Adding cinnamon is one way to trick your palate into thinking you are having something sweet. Eventually you can go to decaffeinated or herbal options later in the day. However, you don't need to cut caffeine out completely. There are recommendations in the appendix for healthier morning caffeine options. As for tea, there are vast selections to choose from, and you will most probably find more than one that you love. A few favorites are white, peach, hibiscus, jasmine, pomegranate, and blueberry green teas. Most teas have less caffeine than coffee and offer us a good option rather than going cold turkey. Eventually, clients are able to cut down on caffeine, and some choose to eliminate it.

Caffeine can negatively affect blood sugar. So transition to keeping caffeinated beverages to the morning. I usually have a black coffee with cinnamon in the morning. Not only does cinnamon taste great, it also helps maintain steady blood sugar levels! In the afternoon, I switch to decaf coffee or decaf green tea. Avoid milk, as both skim and low-fat milk raise blood sugar levels because milk has a naturally occurring sugar called lactose. If you are determined to drink milk, have it at night after dinner. When you drink sugar, you absorb it faster than eating it, which affects blood sugar levels. If you cannot omit dairy in your coffee, go for one tablespoon of heavy cream and skip adding cheese to your next meal. Plain cream has no sugar. Most whipping cream has sugar added. Read labels. Added sugar with caffeine is an even faster way to cause you to crash and burn, so avoid it. It is more satiating to eat your dairy than to drink it. You could choose a small amount of cheese (two tablespoons of parmesan, crumbled blue, or gorgonzola) added to a salad, for example, over cream in coffee.

At the beginning of this book, I said the nutrition part is easy, and it is. Three days on the FAITH VS. WEIGHT diet, and you will have the basic hang of it. Although there are many diets, you will never know if this plan is the winner if you don't give it at least three days. See the testimonials section if you need a boost of faith. Even though you may have doubts, you can succeed on this plan because it is easy and doesn't leave you feeling deprived. Receiving texts from excited clients who share good news from their doctor appointments is exciting for all involved. However, before they did the diet, they put their faith in the Lord Jesus Christ. I hope the same for you, whatever diet you do.

Although this plan was created for the adult female, spouses are getting in on the act, and these men have been making fast strides with this program. Children are addressed in week seven. Each client's plan is different because there are several options. This plan has been tried and tested through multiple focus groups and has been the easiest way for my clients to curb their cravings, improve their blood work, and make their weight loss a reality. See the appendix and study the following three charts: eating timing and tips, breakfast/snack, and lunch/dinner options. Practice the three-day rule following these three charts and see what happens. If you are still a doubting Thomas, keep in mind that all of your cells are constantly being replaced. What you put in your body determines how these cells are being fed and what gene expressions are being turned on or off. After three days, you will start craving healthier foods. You were made to enjoy real food. Give it three days.

Make Your Move

"Get up! Pick up your mat and walk."
—John 5:8 (NIV)

The first few chapters focus on food intake. Later chapters focus more on exercise. In the meantime, get up! Week one is all about movement. You need to move every single day. A diabetic client offered the advice to move for fifteen minutes within thirty minutes of each meal to help control blood sugar. At work, get up and walk to the printer, climb stairs between floors, or take a call while pacing around your office. In subsequent chapters, we will get specific with movement and how it affects weight management. For now, just start moving. If you don't think you have time to exercise, let's talk time.

A Time for Everything

My strategic philosophy on exercise is pay now or pay later. If you don't think you have time now, you are often forced to deal with the repercussions later. Expose the lie in your mind telling you that you are too busy to exercise before it is too late. Think of exercise as a priority or prerequisite in order to save time and money. Let's talk time. Medical appointments, therapy, surgeries, and treatments can take up endless amounts of time. Many of these are the consequences of a poor diet and lack of exercise. So you are going to be spending time either way; you might as well get some benefit out of it.

As you age, if you are not taking steps toward improvement, you will speed down the path of decline. It is painful to watch a person who is forty pounds overweight in physical therapy trying to recover from a knee replacement, wondering how long it will take for them to walk again. We are at a time in our history when we have more of what I term "underuse" injuries. We get up from a couch, make an odd turn or move too quickly in another direction, and wind up with a sprained ankle. This can happen to athletes, but it is happening more and more to sedentary people who are injury prone because of weak muscles.

You have the opportunity to manage your weight today and get stronger to avoid one of these underuse injuries tomorrow. That's a two for one. If you are currently in a recovery situation, you can start with the spiritual and nutrition part of your transformation journey. It will help with your recovery. Having been there, I know this can feel like a constant battle, but be encouraged. Every battle you overcome in the name of Jesus sets you up for a bigger victory glorifying God in the process.

Take a Stand

USE YOUR HEAD

Spend a few bucks and buy a journal with a cute cover on it. Each night you will spend five minutes prayer-writing in this journal. Your bedside journal will contain your nightly letters to God (NLG). Throughout this journey, jot down a few thoughts to leave in God's hands before you peacefully drift off to sleep. Your first journal assignment is to create a statement of praise (SOP). This is a bullet list of what you thought were impossible challenges in your life from which the Lord delivered you! These experiences will remind you of the miracles God has already performed in your life. If you happened to have been born in the United States, this is your first miracle! Your SOP will remind you of all the blessings the Lord has showered upon you. Journaling can help you keep things in their proper perspective. Revisiting old journals will demonstrate the Lord's continued faithfulness in your life.

There are many geniuses that have struggled with weight management, so you are in good company. One of the first things excess weight affects is your self-esteem. Unfortunately, people are constantly judging a book by its cover. Even though you know the only people who count in your life are the ones who see you for who you truly are, it still hurts. Your journal will remind you of what you are capable of when you entrust things to the Lord. It will serve as a confidence builder. Good things happen when you do your best and trust the Lord to take care of the rest. Achieving victory over your weight struggles will just be one more thing to add to the list.

Do not stress about losing weight the first week or even expect it. Your body may go into shock just from eating healthy! This is the opposite of diets where you lose a ton of weight the first week and then slow down. It's better to be underwhelmed the first week but thrilled for a lifetime. Focus instead on your energy. Multiple studies show daily weigh-ins keep people in check. However, obsessing over the scale can actually prevent you from reaching your goal. You can use a scale once a week or pick a piece of clothing you try on weekly to measure your progress, but do not make the scale your god.

Look at weight management as you would the stock market. You want your investments to go in a certain direction. If you stress out because yesterday you ate healthy but gained a pound, then you will get derailed and throw healthy eating out the window. If you pulled your stocks out every time you hit a bump in the market, you would never make any money. Instead, monitor and tweak your status. As you follow this program, you will learn to pay attention to what is working and ditch what is not. Make sure you also pay attention to how you feel as your energy increases throughout this journey. The weight will come off!

AVOID ENEMY TERRITORY

What is the most likely outcome if you have food in your house that derails you? If it is a food you can't have just one of, dump it whether it is sugar or carbs. It doesn't mean you can never have this food again. For now, anything eroding your confidence is an invitation to failure. Food is an inanimate object and not something worth suffering over. When you do go shopping, buy the healthy foods suggested on the breakfast/snack and lunch/dinner charts. Choose what's familiar and comfortable to you from the list. When you are tempted to pick up something that derails you, pick another treat you can manage instead. This is practicing prudence! You only have to pass temptation by once at the grocery store. However, once it is at home, you have to pass by it multiple times a day, which is fine, until it's not. If someone else continues to bring temptation into the house, that is their poison, not yours.

Love Your Neighbor

For week one, during your Bible time, ask God to reveal to you the most effective way for you to take better care of yourself in order to love your neighbor. Then start eating for energy. If you aren't already, start moving. Movement will also help you feel more energetic. Everyone can't do everything, but everyone can do something. Listen to what He specifically calls you to do so that you can stop wasting energy on things that are not necessary. Eventually, you will be obeying the command to love your neighbor, because of your newfound energy.

CHANGE YOUR LIFE

Week One: Prudence

I, wisdom, have made prudence my dwelling.
—*Proverbs 8:12 (WEB)*

For Your Soul

Which future is it going to be?

Begin your day with the Lord: Awake, hydrate, and commit to spending at least five minutes in the presence of the Lord. Next, do what Jesus did when the devil tempted Him in the desert with food. Put the Word of God between you and it.

End your day with the Lord. Commit to at least five minutes. Have your journal by your bed for your nightly letter to God (NLG). Over the next week, pick three different nights to commit to completing one of these five minute exercises:

Statement of praise (SOP): jot down all of the accomplishments the Lord has allowed through you and thank Him. He has done it before, and He can do it again.

Strategic outlook: Jot down your strategic outlook, which is "why" you want more energy. If you doubt you can lose the weight, turn the page, and write a letter of encouragement to yourself as if you were writing it to a friend. Be your own biggest fan and address each area of doubt. You have to learn to love yourself if you are going to love your neighbor.

Look up a Bible verse that supports your strategic outlook.

Add your Bible quote as a daily reminder on your phone.

This is a journey. Walk with the Lord.

For Your Body

Practice prudence by asking yourself, "What is the most likely outcome of what I am about to do?" *before* you do it. Is what you are about to eat or drink going to give you more energy or suck the life out of you?

Take a picture of the FAITH VS. WEIGHT Diet in the appendix.

For now, you only need to focus on the charts in the appendix. Print and copy: eating timing and tips; breakfast/snack; and lunch/dinner charts. Put them on your fridge, on your phone, and so on.

Pick the foods you like from the FAITH VS. WEIGHT Diet.

Go shopping.

Eat for energy: commit to doing the plan for three days.

Get up and move within thirty minutes of eating with a goal of fifteen minutes of movement. This may be as simple as making a phone call while walking around your desk.

Avoid enemy territory: get rid of any food that tempts you to overeat. It doesn't mean goodbye forever, but for now, you are committing to failure if you keep it in the house. It's not worth eroding your self-confidence over.

Separate junk food from healthy food. If you live with other people who eat cookies and candies, have a separate drawer for their stuff. You do not need to be harassed by a cookie gauntlet on your way to grab your hundred-calorie pistachios.

Reminder: no one has changed with just this diet alone. If giving you a diet made you skinny, we'd all be skinny! The reason you are choosing this diet makes all the difference. As you commit to follow the suggestions in each chapter, you better your chances of long-term success.

Temperance

And everyone who competes for the prize is temperate in all things. Now they do it to obtain a perishable crown, but we for an imperishable crown.

—1 Corinthians 9:25 (NKJV)

Rarely do you hear someone bragging about how much temperance (self-control) they have. Most people struggle in this area. Our problem with self-control is our tendency to focus on the "self" part of self-control instead of the prize we attain by exercising it. Even if we are smart enough to focus on the prize instead of our own struggles, the prize has to be worth it. Paul and other believers were excited about striving in order to receive an "imperishable crown." Even though the prize was not easily attainable, they did not focus on the struggle. They focused on the prize. The more excited you are about your prize, the less power self and all of its struggles will have over you.

This chapter focuses on the prize, because the rewards of self-control eventually diminish the need for it. When temperance becomes a habit in a certain area, it no longer feels like self-control. It's just another habit. First, we are going to look at temperance from the perspective of an athlete preparing for a race. Second, we will explore how other cultures traditionally approach temperance as a way of life. In both cases, self-control is just a means to an end that has become a habit. The end is the prize. In the case of the athlete, the prize is to win. In the case of traditional cultural practices, the prize it is to behave in a way supported and valued in that culture. Finally, you will learn practical tips from both perspectives that will set you on a path for victory.

THE WHITE HOUSE

As a White House Military Social Aide, representing the Navy, I had the honor of assisting with event execution at medal of honor ceremonies, state dinners, and Christmas events. Many of these were decadent affairs. Yet the White House was the first place I remember noticing temperance in action. One late evening, I was surprised to see a navy aide pass up various desserts after a state dinner, made by the White House chefs. With less than 7 percent body fat, this aide could have afforded a truffle (or ten), but he had his eyes on a different prize. He competed in half-ironman triathlons and was not interested in anything that might slow him down for his upcoming race. The Bible verse above referred to a race—think Olympics. Since this aide was not competing in the Olympics, I was in awe that he would actually pass up a dessert made by a White House chef. What prize could be worth that level of self-denial? I wondered this as I also wondered if there were any truffle flavors I had accidentally missed.

Another noticeable thing about this navy aide was that he did not appear to look deprived. As a matter of fact, he actually seemed elated! He couldn't wait to get up at 5:00 the next morning to drive for hours to compete in yet another half-ironman. At the time, I considered a fast walk to the metro a workout and could not comprehend going through that kind of effort to win a medal. Oddly enough, he wasn't even into medals! The prize he was seeking was not the medal but achieving his personal best (PB). This is a term used to describe an athlete's best performance to date. Everyone wants to win first place, but he concentrated on striving for first place based on his own performance. He didn't even necessarily pick the races he could win! He purposely ran with people who were faster than him. What drives people to do this?

To unearth the answer, I had to go to great lengths. I had to marry him (the things people will do to write a book). Eventually, I learned his secret, the secret of all athletes, and the secret contained in the above Bible verse.

The secret to self-control has nothing to do with self-control but has everything to do with the prize you are seeking and what you perceive its value to be. Are you in love with your prize or not?

For athletes to have a chance at victory, they have to exercise an inordinate amount of self-control. They have to train when they don't feel like training and say no to foods when they don't feel like saying no. They have to do this every day, and in some cases for hours a day! They exercise self-control by choice because they love competing. They strive for first place even though their best effort may not be enough. Striving is not an "all or nothing" event; it is a consistent measured effort toward an athlete's personal best. Athletes remain on this journey even though they have no guarantee of winning a perishable crown. The imperishable crown the believers referenced in the above verse is striving for a PB for the glory of God. Their prize was doing their personal best for Jesus.

In order for you to be at your personal best, you also need to employ temperance. Temperance creates energy by not wasting it. Athletes have to conserve lots of energy in order to be able to exert lots of energy, and so do you. You can't afford to waste your energy on lesser things. Temperance and energy are a type of ying and yang that feed off each other in a positive way. Since the goal is not to waste energy, there are two main ways we need to be mindful in order to avoid squandering energy (other than unhealthy food and a lack of exercise). First, your PB is going to look a lot different from someone else's. That doesn't matter. Just stay in your lane. Go for your PB or you will waste energy worrying about everyone else's and throw temperance along with your potential out the window. This is not called NB—your neighbor's best. This is called PB, your personal best. Too many people get caught up in the comparison trap and lose the race, along with other opportunities to win, before they even enter. Instead, conserve your energy by keeping your eyes on your prize, like a racehorse with blinders on ...

Don't turn from it to the right hand or to the left, that you may have good success wherever you go.

—*Joshua 1:7 (WEB)*

Second, the more you value (love) your prize, the more energy you will invest in seeking it. If your "why" does not feel as if it is a prize worth fighting for, you are going to waste a lot of energy on cheap imitations. Is your why bigger than a doughnut? If it isn't, ask the Lord to direct you to verses in the Bible to help you fall in love with your why. If your why is from the Lord, it will be your heart's desire. This desire He places in your heart is where your why lives. The above Bible verse written by Paul describes his why. Temperance was just a means to an end in order to achieve it. The imperishable crown he writes about is one of the five crowns mentioned earlier as a reward for believers. This particular crown is the prize for those who have led a temperate life. In order to achieve this, Paul kept his eyes on the prize of becoming more like Christ, not his unending struggles. Hopefully, with each new day, we are heading in that same direction.

Love the Lord Your God

Do you believe it is impossible for you to practice temperance when it comes to food? Ask yourself if you are answering this question based on your current beliefs about your self-control or as if God is in control. If the prize you are seeking is your God-given heart's desire, then God has already equipped you with all of the self-control you will ever need to attain it. Once you are born again, you are already a contender for the imperishable crown!

> *For you have been born again, not from perishable seed, but imperishable, through the word of God which lives and abides forever.*
>
> *—1 Peter 1:23 (MEV)*

The imperishable seed has been planted in all believers, including you! It is already alive in you. Without self-control, you would probably not have a job, an education, or a spouse. Nor would you have very many friends over the long haul. Victories in all areas of your life would be few and far between. Yet in the US, an all-or-nothing mentality, the opposite of temperance, is celebrated. Denying yourself because you are striving for a prize is quite different from denying yourself because you think you should be denying yourself. Unfortunately, the latter is how most people view healthy eating. In the first case, you are excited about the prize, but in the second, you are already set up to fail. Self-control is all how you look at it. Everyone thinks they have to have more self-control in order to follow Jesus, when the opposite is true. We need Jesus in order to have self-control. This is a supernatural power you do not have without Him. Self-control in all areas can sound overwhelming, but in reality, there is only one area where you need self-control, and that is in deciding how close you are willing to walk with Jesus. The closer you walk with Jesus, the more temperate you will be in all things, because now you are putting God in control instead of self. You are not interested in anything that comes between the two of you. As soon as you realize He alone can fill your needs, you outgrow them. Therein lies your self-control.

Therefore if anyone is in Christ, he is a new creation. The old things
have passed away. Behold, all things have become new.

—2 Corinthians 5:17 (WEB)

BACK TO THE GARDEN

My guess is Eve was not walking around the Garden of Eden the day the
devil tempted her thinking, *Gee, I want to be just like God.* She was just
enjoying the garden when the devil tempted her to believe God was holding
out on her. The devil wants you to believe that God is holding out on you
also. God is the one spoiling all of the fun. This ignores the fact that God
actually created fun and had placed Eve in Eden. Regardless, the devil easily
convinced Eve God was denying something to which she felt entitled. Do
you have an entitlement mentality? Since pride is the root of all evil, it is easy
to fall into this trap. Knowing this, the devil then asked, "Has God really
said, 'You shall not eat of any tree of the garden?'" —Genesis 3:1 (WEB).

Newsflash: Satan already knew the answer and was creating doubt. He is
asking you a similar question, "Is this nutty lady really trying to convince
you that you can actually have more self-control? It's not going to happen."
We don't like it when we have a perceived need and someone keeps us from
satisfying it. We don't want to miss out! Besides, we convince ourselves that
we deserve that extra cookie because it's been a stressful day.

For God knows that in the day you eat it, your eyes will be opened,
and you will be like God.

—Genesis 3:5 (WEB)

Who doesn't want to be just like God since God can do whatever He wants!
No one wants to be told what she can and cannot do. This is called pride.
Turning your life over to Jesus is saying, "Jesus, I trust you to be the Lord of
my life. I will follow you, even when I don't *feel* like it." This is about saying
no to any excess that steals your energy to follow Him. Following Christ is
putting your pride, including impulsive wants, aside so you are game for
whatever is next on His agenda for your life. This requires self-control. That

doesn't sound like much fun, because it isn't, unless you are more focused on the prize than the struggle. Satan wants to keep you focused on your struggles. The Lord wants to keep you focused on His glory, because that is what is going to lead you to eternal victory. This is much better than following Satan's lies that appear to fulfill an immediate need today but instead only create more want tomorrow. He whispers, "Yes, you deserve that sea salt caramel. Your electrolytes must be low. Why don't you have extra whip while you're at it?"

Change Your Brain

You don't have to participate in the same level of self-denial as an athlete, but you do have to exert a sustained effort. Without it, victories are few and far between. Contrary to popular belief, a sustained effort is actually a lot easier than all or nothing. Many people all over the world apply a sustained effort without knowing it because it has become a habit. This is the goal. However, in the US, our tendency is to either obsess over or ignore our habits. Neither approach is conducive to temperance. The good news is you are not born with your habits. Just as you learned your habits, you can unlearn them. As you visualize your prize, you will be inspired to replace self-defeating habits with ones that lead to victory.

Bon Appetit!

Many cultures around the world practice temperance with their tradition-al eating habits. They eat a certain way without even thinking about it. Temperance is a part of their cultural norm, so it has become a habit; this is not so in the United States. It's time to take a vacation from all or nothing.

Let's zip on over on our Vespa to an outdoor café in Paris I once visited. It was a starlit evening with most Parisians looking as if they had just left a French *Vogue* photo shoot (not a whole lot of sweatpants here). The women were rather petite compared to American standards. They probably had never even seen the inside of a gym or tried the latest fad diet. At last it was finally time for dessert, and the table next to ours was about to order. I couldn't wait to see what was on the menu!

Wait a minute? Did I hear that right? Did she just order? This must have been a language barrier thing. Oh my goodness, it actually looked like … was it really … a piece of … fruit? *Seriously*? She ordered one slice of cantaloupe. Are you kidding? Doesn't she know this is a culinary capital of the world? On top of that, she was eating it with a fork and knife. I had never seen anyone eat a cantaloupe with a fork and a knife. Sorry, I must not have gotten out much! I mean, maybe if the cantaloupe was cut up in a fruit salad, I might have eaten it with a fork. Anyway, she savored her "dessert" as if it were some sort of sumptuous delicacy!

Her friend ordered mini cakes called petit fours. At least this woman was not going to disappoint! Well, they were a little small (a square inch), but this was France. At least this was actually a real dessert. However, after a bite or two, she appeared disinterested. Was there something wrong with her dessert? Did she want something else instead? Wasn't she worried about wasting her food? Apparently, she did not subscribe to this way of thinking. She certainly was not a member of the "clean your plate" club!

The two French women continued to sip their coffee, chatting and laughing while admiring the starry night. It seemed like they were more interested in enjoying the ambience of the evening than getting their money's worth by licking their plate clean. Then it was time to go. Was something actually more interesting than their dessert?

This was another example of people being prudent or temperate with dessert and still appearing to be happy! Is being happy with having either no dessert or a small amount a foreign concept to you? I had only seen people (present company included) miserable, claiming they were on a diet, giving up dessert as if it were a fate worse than death, or overdoing it. Yet these two women got up from their dinner, looking just as good as when they walked in, ending with a stroll down the Avenue des Champs Elysées. I guess they had better things to do.

I am thankful that the US has taken major steps to educate the public on healthy eating, but I am afraid going for a stroll on a starry night in lieu of overdoing dessert is a thing of the past. Unfortunately, you are more likely to find us with a gargantuan plate of nachos supreme at a restaurant before our main course has even been ordered, let alone dessert. If not, we may be gulping down pizza, fast food, or a bag of "30 percent more free" of some unidentifiable ingredients while lounging in our expandable sweatpants in a semi-comatose media trance. Last time I checked, that's not why Jesus came.

I am not saying you should move to France (although I do enjoy visiting). This was just where I happened to be when I first noticed temperance practiced as part of a cultural lifestyle. Since then, I have also seen temperance practiced in Japan, Spain, Austria, Prague, Italy, Israel, and Switzerland. Temperance is probably the reason why the French, Japanese, and Swiss women are not fat when they follow their traditional diet. This sounds like a gross generalization, but these countries have lower obesity rates. Temperance is practiced and celebrated within traditional diets in these cultures. It has become a habit.

These cultures have another easy-to-overlook practice in common. They all end their meals with coffee or tea. My unscientific theory (until someone proves it) is these beverages, with no sugar added, are a consistent cue to the brain to stop eating. I have experimented with this concept with decaf and herbal teas, and it works. You don't need a double-shot expresso. It may be that coffee and tea (without sugar) have a more acidic taste that triggers the brain to stop eating. If you add sugar, I don't find the same effect. Without sugar, and even with a touch of cinnamon in your coffee and tea, you may have the ying to the sugar yang. This simple move has cut through my sugar cravings like a knife. Why not carry white, herbal, or decaf green tea bags with you to dinner functions? Have it with a piece of dark chocolate instead of plowing into a towering dessert that will keep you up all night. Hot beverages without sugar also tend to slow you down when you eat dessert.

As you would imagine, these cultures typically have a small amount of coffee or tea. You don't need the 24-ounce mega size. Four to six ounces is plenty with an equally small dessert. Although it would be wonderful to also see everyone take a walk after dinner, it seems to be just as unrealistic to suggest we eat slower. However, both are huge factors within these cultures. When you eat quickly, you eat more. If you are going to have a dessert, have a small amount and *savor* it, instead of inhaling it in a trance at the checkout line. Studies show people are no more satisfied after the third bite whether they have three bites or twenty. However, they are extremely dissatisfied when they cannot fit into their pants.

What Has Food Done for You Lately?

Successful advertisements for chocolate products, especially around Valentine's Day, are designed to create an emotional response. Of course the women in these commercials are all skinny and gorgeous—a little different from the rest of us. On top of that, their adoringly perfect husbands picked out those chocolate confections for them. We want to be just like them! Look, they can eat a particular brand of chocolate and still be skinny! Why can't we? So we use food to stuff down our emotions and live the marketer's dream. We are just happy we got it at 50 percent off! Although somehow, we are not savoring it and eating "just one" like the supermodel lookalike in the commercial.

An emotional response to food is one of the number one reasons many struggle with temperance. Just like you have a need for love, you also have a need for nourishment, and both needs can be satisfied in life-giving ways. In your search for love, you may wind up looking for it in all of the wrong places, leaving you even lonelier than when you started. This creates more doubt in your ability to have a healthy relationship with yourself and others. Many struggling with their weight feel as if they are not quite up to par, doubting they will ever find peace with their body or food again. Maybe you would never put up with this abuse from another person. No way. You have way too much going for you than to put up with that kind of abuse from anybody—except, of course, from yourself. Instead, give yourself some grace.

Your destiny hinges on whether or not you choose to look into your Father's eyes, the only one capable of satisfying your hungry heart, or do what most people do, and look out. If you look away from God, you will always be looking. The search for love or avoiding pain is the cause of many addictions. Addictions are the opposite of temperance. Unfortunately, most people prefer to look for a quick fix, only to make things worse, until they are distracted by the next quick fix. There are plenty of enticements, including all types of advertisements vying to sell you the next quick fix, disguised as love, in order to create an emotional response to a product. Because we are so isolated, this may be the most emotional connection some of us get all day.

The key here is to change the object of your affection. A box of chocolates is never going to seem like a good idea the morning after. However, happy, healthy relationships do exist! I want you to look at your relationship with food in the same way. It's never too late, but you need to look up instead of out. Once you look up, you may be guided to get help in other areas of your life holding you back. Oftentimes counseling in one area cures a problem in another. Food is an inanimate object. It is neither bad nor good. How we use it determines whether or not it is giving us energy or sucking the life out of us.

> *Do not be anxious about anything, but in every situation, by prayer and petition, with thanksgiving, present your requests to God. And the peace of God, which transcends all understanding, will guard your hearts and your minds in Christ Jesus.*
>
> *—Philippians 4:6–7 (NIV)*

The first verse tells you to stop worrying and ask God for what you need, including love. The second verse tells you He will give you a peace so great you cannot even comprehend it because the Lord Jesus Christ is guarding your heart. In other words, you already asked, so trust God to take care of it because you cannot begin to understand the way in which He will answer your request. Stop wasting your energy by trying to take things back into your own hands or trying to figure out what you can't understand. Trust the Almighty God who is guarding your heart, the heart He made, to take care of it in His way. Do you think anyone else, including you, can do a better job? He's got this.

Eat for Energy

One of the number one things I tell my clients about temperance, whether it is at home, at a restaurant, or at a celebration, is: this is not the Last Supper. Unless of course it is your last day on the planet, then I believe shortly you will be more excited about things other than brownies on the other side of the pearly gates. Another thing to keep in mind is an Italian quote, "Anche l'occhio vuole la sua parte," translated: "The eye wants its share too." Eat the rainbow. Food looks prettier, tastes better, and is better for you when you include more vegetables. You will feel more satisfied and less tempted to overdo it. One of the reasons you may overeat is because you are eating foods of negligible nutritional value. Most things that come in a bag or box are lacking. If you want to learn how to be temperate, you need to eat real food. You have practically unlimited options. It is easier to be temperate when you are receiving proper nourishment and eating real food that looks good. Salad bars are one of the easiest ways to do this without cooking. Just make sure you add protein and healthy fat. You can also buy different frozen veggies and steam or microwave them, including riced and shredded versions. Originally, people were having riced cauliflower to replace rice, but you can also enjoy riced Brussels sprouts or broccoli. These vegetables are delicious with extra virgin olive oil and a touch of iodized sea salt added once they are cooked.

IT'S ALL GREEK TO ME

The Sirens in Greek mythology used to lure sailors with their enchanting music and beauty, only to have them crash along the rocky coast. These Sirens held the promise of something that would satisfy human desire but instead destroyed the seeker. Among other things, this luring reminds me of our processed food supply. Every day, there is yet another new candy, cookie, drink, or some other confection luring you in. What about asking yourself whether or not something with an undetermined shelf life and a list of ingredients requiring a toxicologist to decipher can actually be good for you?

Guess what? Your body doesn't have a PhD either. This is part of the reason many diets fail. Most diets are not sustainable because they do not provide enough nutrient-dense calories (we are starving), and they are loaded with processed foods (we are taking in chemicals), triggering cravings. Processed foods are slowly killing America with very few exceptions. Most are created so you will never be satisfied.

> *You have planted much but harvest little. You eat but are not satisfied.*
> *You drink but are still thirsty.*
>
> *—Haggai 1:6 (NLT)*

Never being satisfied is personified in the Greek mythology character Tantalus. You have probably already guessed his name is the origin for the word "tantalize." Suffering from extreme pride, he wanted to show he was the greatest by outsmarting all of the Greek gods but got caught in the act. Furious, Zeus (his father) was not quite satisfied with just killing Tantalus, so he decided to put him in an eternal state of not being satisfied. Tantalus suffered from eternal hunger and eternal thirst. Every time he tried to get close to the dangling fruit or water nearby, they moved farther away. This reminds me of what food manufacturers call the bliss point. The bliss point in food manufacturing is the amount of sugar, salt, and fat, or their substitutes added to make something irresistible or almost impossible to eat "just one." This also applies to the coffee industry. Gourmet coffees are loaded with chemicals. Unfortunately, most coffees have the same (or more) calories as an ice-cream shake, or they are completely loaded with fake sugars, which are unable to ever satisfy cravings.

There is nothing wrong with you. Your body chemistry, which is influenced by a myriad of factors beyond genetics, may make it harder for you than someone else to eat or drink just one. Some can have one glass of wine, whereas someone else may evolve into an alcoholic. Likewise, it is more difficult for some than others to minimize sugar and its substitutes. In this case, it is even harder for some people than resisting alcohol, since sugar is ubiquitous and not only socially accepted but also celebrated. We haven't figured out yet that the overconsumption of processed foods and sugar is actually killing us, so many of us are in an eternal state of buying. Just like

Tantalus, you will never be satisfied. Eventually, you may feel like you have had enough for one day but not without cost. A client shared with me about a friend who was going to counseling for a crack addiction. She told me the counselor would say the following words over and over again, "You are still searching for that first hit." I can't think of a better way to put it. The Sirens and Tantalus remind us that Satan puts out the best first, only to leave us wanting in the end, left with the worst.

From a spiritual standpoint, when you use and then later abuse people or things for a purpose other than what God intended, you will also wind up crashing on a rocky coast. It usually does not appear this way in the beginning. Similar to the call of the Sirens, these situations appear wonderfully enticing. Of course they do, or why else would we be game? It even looks like something you have under control. Yet it can escalate into something you do not recognize, causing you to no longer recognize yourself. God doesn't give you self-control so you can have a boring life. He gives you temperance to protect you so that you can have fullness of life.

DISORDERED EATING OR EATING DISORDER

Eating disorders require professional help. However, the majority of overeating is not necessarily tied to an eating disorder. Sugar, chemicals, exhaustion, and stress are all linked to overeating. If I start the day with sugar, the rest of the day winds up being a train wreck. Keep sugar as a dessert, and no earlier, other than the honey in the pre-workout drink suggested. (See eating timing and tips.) If you consume sugar earlier in the day, you will have problems with portion control all day. Throw in some emotional drama, and it can be the difference between having one ice-cream cone or an all-out bender. So how do you know if you have a problem requiring medical intervention?

The first place to look to determine whether or not you need outside help is your trigger foods. Most people are not binge eating celery. Many snack foods are trigger foods. They tempt you without ever satisfying you. Many of the "healthy" packaged options lead to more overeating. Real food that is not processed gives your body all the right signals to cue satiation. However, even with real food, you can get your signals crossed. Cut out processed foods first to see if you still have a problem. Then pay attention to which real foods leave you feeling satiated and full for hours or looking for a way to break into the vending machine. Sugar, starchy carbohydrates, salt, and fat can all trigger cravings. Another trigger is hunger. If you are starving, you are less likely to stop at an appropriate amount. Again, starving equals stuffed. You need to eat at regular intervals. Follow the eating timing and tips chart. If you are in a bind, at least have a hundred-calorie pack of nuts, dried edamame, or pistachios in the shell on hand as an emergency snack.

The hypothalamus is the part of the brain controlling hunger. If you are eating regularly and are cued by legitimate hunger before you start a balanced meal and not by habit, boredom, lack of sleep, emotions, or stale cookies left out in the breakroom, you will also be cued when you are full and satiated. How do you feel after a meal containing real food versus junk? Studies show people report less satisfaction after snacks than meals, which makes perfect sense since most people are eating junk for snacks, or their snacks are not enough calories, causing them to want to graze all day. This is why we include a substantial snack such as nuts/nut butter or edamame in our afternoon snack with fruit instead of fruit alone. A snack should be adequate enough to get your mind off food without ruining your appetite for your next meal. Food is meant to fortify and satisfy in order to make you stop thinking about food and begin the task at hand. Eating is not meant to serve as an ongoing entertainment, hobby, or distraction. It is meant to keep you fueled.

On that note, if you need a morning snack and are skipping it because you typically eat an early lunch, you can have your morning snack a couple of hours after your lunch and then have your afternoon snack later in the day before dinner. Many of my clients who are teachers do this because they have to eat early lunches and do not have time for a morning snack before lunch, so they have it a couple of hours after lunch. It they don't push their morning snack to early afternoon while also having their afternoon snack later in the day, they wind up starving by dinner.

SPECIAL OCCASION OR NOT

I love to celebrate! However, the term "special occasion" makes me cringe. Why? Temperance seems to go out the window. Endless streams of new clients overdo it on special occasions. As mentioned, I never subscribe to the guilt philosophy. I just ask clients how they felt after the indulgence. In case you were wondering, it is the same answer for a special occasion as it is for a regular occasion. Sugar is still sugar even if it is a special occasion. It's important to remember how you feel after the party is over. Then it's time to mentally rehearse a more favorable outcome, like an athlete going over a play to prepare for future success. Otherwise, special occasions result in our feeling not so special! If this were only once in a while, it would be no big deal, but we each must have at least ten special occasions a month in the US. Let's see … we have a coworker's baby shower, an anniversary, a birthday party, and then another birthday party. Then we have Boss's Day, Secretary's Day, Teacher Appreciation Day, Sibling's Day, Mother's Day, Father's Day, Grandparents' Day, and Mother's-in-Law Day (didn't even realize this one existed until recently). We have company in and out of town. Notice I have not even mentioned a single holiday between Halloween and Valentine's Day or the Fourth of July barbecues. "On and on it goes, and where it stops, nobody knows." You may love to celebrate! However, you do not need to overeat for everyone else's special occasion. A card, flowers, or some balloons can make it special. Overeating does not make it special. Besides designated special occasions, it is a rare occasion when I don't hear someone say they need to lose weight after a recent vacation. It is also common to hear people talking about how they overdid it at a restaurant or at a function on an ordinary day. Special occasions, vacations, and restaurant visits do not have to equal weight gain! There is definitely a correlation but no causation.

I have helped many clients continue to lose weight over the holidays. Because of this, I was recently asked to present holiday eating tips before a group of seventy women. I told them I count only seven days between Halloween and Valentine's Day of which most Americans celebrate as a holiday. (This does not include every holiday or every religious celebration. One can insert their religious holiday/festival in place of the others listed.) The point here is there are only seven days between Halloween and Valentine's that are actually considered holidays. We are looking at the following: Halloween (or fall festival), Thanksgiving, Christmas Eve, Christmas Day, New Year's Eve, New Year's Day, and Valentine's Day. Only seven days between October 31 and Febraury14 of overdoing it are probably not going to cause you to sell the farm! The problem is we are also overdoing it all of the other days during this four-month span. Basically one-third of the year is spent overeating under the guise of the holidays! Not just at parties but all of the time. Not getting a handle on overeating at the holidays is like a snowball rolling downhill, increasing in size and mass each year.

My friend Jane calls the holidays the "eating season." She and her husband joke that they actually have to train the rest of the year to get ready for it. One of the tips I gave to this particular group of women I spoke with was not to buy Halloween candy before Halloween. Halloween candy is now on the shelves starting September 1. We are talking a full sixty days of eating before the actual holiday. I promise you this: stores sell plenty of Halloween candy during those sixty days. However, when October 31 rolled around, and we bought our candy, there was still plenty on the shelves. Today is the day before Thanksgiving, and every place I stopped had huge bowls of Halloween candy right out on their front desk, or maybe they just have it out year-round, and I hadn't noticed. If it is not an actual holiday, you don't need to eat as if it is.

Even during the holiday season, most of your breakfasts, lunches, snacks, and dinners are completely up to you. Don't blow your calories on boring everyday stuff you don't really love. Continue to maintain a healthy diet and save your hundred-calorie treat allowance for a childhood favorite or a gourmet dessert at a holiday party. With desserts, ask yourself after the first bite if what you are eating is calorie worthy before inhaling something you weren't even crazy about in the first place. Just because it is there and has sugar in it doesn't mean it is your favorite. I was not born doing this, and I learned to do it. I teach my clients the same thing, and they learned to do it. This is just about awareness. Ask yourself if what you are eating is worth wearing on your trouble areas because this is exactly where it is going! It is not a lot of fun to save for a special holiday dress and not be able to fit into it. More importantly, ask yourself if whatever you are eating is giving you energy to enjoy all of this holiday fun or making you miserable because you keep overdoing it. Is this behavior getting you closer to your prize or farther away? If you are tempted to overdo it, just remember how we started this section. *This is not the Last Supper!* You will have another dessert tomorrow, and the day after and the day after that, because this plan allows for a dessert every single day. Just pick a holiday item for your dessert or pick one of the options suggested on the lunch/dinner chart in the appendix. I have not had a single client who could not find something that worked for them. You can do it.

We also need to avoid the all-or-nothing mentality eating the day of an event. I hear people say all the time they "eat light" before going to a holiday function. I cannot think of a better recipe for disaster unless you are a naturally thin person. I suggest the total opposite. I tell clients not to go to any event starving. I eat all day before an event … the same amount I eat every single day. I treat the event dinner the same way I do every other dinner. No reason to overdo it. If you go starving, you will leave stuffed. Over time, the health implications of this go beyond the scale. It's just a dinner, not a reason to give up on your dreams. Enjoy the reason you are actually going: the company.

In most cases, the problem is actually not your holiday favorite but the amount. If your holiday favorite is something you cannot be temperate with, even after being on this plan, ditch it for now. This is actually a great way to figure out if something works in your life. You either learn to have a small amount for dessert or you get rid of it. It is entirely up to you. There really is not a third option unless you want to crash and burn. For some reason, we feel since it is the holidays we need to gobble up as much as we can as fast as we can. If you have a holiday favorite that you tend to overdo because you fear it is only available once a year, there are two ways to combat this. Have a little and save the rest for the next day. You can enjoy it over more days! You can also buy or make more of whatever this favorite item is at any other time of the year. We pretty much have this option in the USA. However, my guess is there will be another dessert looking even more interesting at that point. You can also remind yourself there will be plenty more treats to eat over the holidays. Tomorrow will be another day, so space it out. Something better will come along. Think abundance, not scarcity. Of the near-death experiences I have read about, no one has mentioned regret over not having more desserts.

Although we blame overeating on the holidays, in many cases, we are longing for something food is not going to satisfy. Take a step back and ask yourself what you are trying to replace with food. It may be the memory of a loved one. They are in your heart. It may be the fact you are still single or recently divorced. The Christmas cookie is not going to help you with this either. I know because I have been in both of these categories, mourning over the loss of a loved one, and being one of the only singles party after party, long after my friends were having their second or third child. I also remember what Christmas was like after my parents were divorced.

As benign as this may sound, start singing some Christmas carols and redirect. Worship music has helped many redirect through a crisis and can allow you to share the joy of Christ with others. Many years ago, I lost my father to a tragic accident two days before Christmas. I know how it feels. I also know Jesus came, and Christmas is a time to celebrate the King of kings, so I focus on this aspect every year and know my father is with Him. Do not let the devil steal your joy! Celebrate instead of fixate. Christmas carols can help a great deal in this area celebrating our Savior! Sign up to go caroling at a senior facility or hospital. Sign up to serve food at a homeless shelter. Just sign up. There is plenty of need everywhere. Fill up on sharing the love of Christ, not the eggnog.

Bon Voyage

At the mention of vacation, the word *recreation* comes to mind, with the root word being create, or recreate. Why go on a vacation only to come back to work that has piled up and the additional burden of weight gain? Since vacations equal restaurant eating, we are now going to cover your best strategies for restaurants. Your best strategy starts before you even get to the restaurant. First, hydrate, hydrate, hydrate. Second, don't forget snacks on vacation. You need your snacks on vacation just like you do when you are not on vacation.

If you don't snack as suggested on the FAITH VS. WEIGHT diet, you will arrive at your vacation dinners starving. Again, *starving equals stuffed.* Do not forget healthy snacks. You can get hundred-calorie nuts through airport security. You can also usually find an apple somewhere in an airport to have with your hundred-calories nuts. Pack raw cacao and coconut packs so you can have naturally sugar-free hot cacao while traveling. This doesn't take much extra space. This just takes planning ahead. If you want to feel just as good when you come back from your vacation as you did before you left, plan ahead. It is a wonderful feeling to come home energized from a vacation instead of bloated. Planning for a few minutes each day and before trips can save you forty to fifty pounds over a year.

RESTAURANTS

When you first arrive at a restaurant, always drink water. Then order a salad or raw vegetable appetizer. Why? Because by the time the restaurant brings the main course, everyone is usually starving, and the table has already ordered an appetizer. Even if you had the virtuous intention of a grilled salmon salad with avocado as your main course, by now you have eaten the bread basket and plowed into the gooey, fatty appetizer equaling twice as many calories than what you had planned. Instead, order a salad, crudités, veggie plate, or broth-based soup as your appetizer. I will even order a garden salad as an appetizer if my entrée is going to be a grilled protein with salad. More vegetables have yet to kill anyone. Have your appetizer veggies with a healthy fat like olive oil, olives, guacamole, hummus, or two tablespoons of nuts on the side. This will count as your fat serving. Enjoy your entrée with two tablespoons of cheese that you ordered on the side. This simple appetizer and entrée trick can save you thousands of calories over a month's time. When I am at restaurants, people comment that I have lots of willpower. I do not. What I do have is the FAITH VS. WEIGHT Diet plan that I am teaching you. By following it, I avoid putting myself in situations where I am starving, making it much easier to make temperate decisions.

What about a glass of wine? The FAITH VS. WEIGHT motto on alcohol is "one or none." Dementia and Alzheimer's are on the rise, and they do not respond well to alcohol since alcohol is poison for your brain. Besides a high sugar diet, excess alcohol is another one of your brain's worst enemies. Most people who drink tend to either overeat or overdrink, and the overeating is not excess vegetables. It is easy to lose track of calories when alcohol is involved. If you want the Resveratrol, give yourself a serving of grapes after dinner instead! If you are committed to having one glass of wine, then have one glass of wine. The problem is I don't see many people sticking with one. Although we hear a lot about opiate abuse, alcohol abuse is also on the rise for women.

I had an older client who was on a fixed income wanting to drink one glass of wine with her meals. However, she always wound up having two. She did not want to give up on the idea of having one glass, even though she knew she was overdoing it. Instead of forfeiting the ability to help her, we tried something called harm reduction, which is basically reducing the amount. Much of the FAITH VS. WEIGHT Diet is based on this theory. I told her to buy the most expensive glass she could afford and sip it slowly. Since she was on a fixed income, this actually was a big deal for her. I also told her to have water on the table since alcohol dehydrates. She was happy with this outcome. Even though in her mind she was "losing" a second glass of wine, she was "gaining" the reward of a higher-quality glass of wine. I suggest the same thing when I have people switch to higher quality chocolate instead of the stuff that has an indefinite shelf life while also being NASA approved for space orbit. I am not recommending alcohol, but if you are going to drink it, the rule for this plan is "one or none." Decide if prudence or temperance is the right answer for you. Alcohol is not worth God's glory.

ENTERTAINING

When I entertain, I always offer healthy options. Home is the easiest environment to control. For appetizers, I serve raw veggies with hummus or guacamole. For drinks, we have unsweetened teas or sparkling/filtered water with cucumber or lemon and orange slices. In the summer, we usually have barbecues offering a couple of protein options for the main meal, and a dinner vegetable like steamed asparagus or my personal favorite, vegetable shish kabobs. These are always a big hit because they look fancy, taste delicious, and require no prep since most grocery stores offer these premade in the summer. I also always have a carb option for my guests. It may be bean salad, brown rice, or gluten-free buns if we are having turkey or grass-fed beef burgers. My guests are happy to bring dessert because then everyone gets exactly what they want. Stick with a small piece and savor it with a glass of unsweetened tea in the summer or hot herbal tea in the winter.

Being Entertained

I have known clients who previously did not attend holiday parties or go to restaurants out of fear of overdoing it. Others decide to go but still have anxiety about overeating since they are trying to lose weight or maybe have made some progress and are afraid to derail it. Anyone who has tried to lose weight understands. However, the problem with this thinking is we are meant for fellowship. Avoiding an ice-cream joint on your way home every day makes sense. Giving up social activities you love with good friends does not. When I am a guest, I offer to bring raw veggies and hummus or guacamole (veggies and a healthy fat). If I know I am going somewhere that is only going to have pizza (let's say a kid party), I will also bring a protein. Shrimp cocktail from the grocery store for the adults is a zero-cook protein and is always a hit. As of yet, no host has been disappointed when I have shown up with shrimp cocktail!

When being entertained, it is natural for someone to offer you different foods. When someone says to me, "Oh you should try the _____," and it is something I do not plan on having, I just smile and say, "Thank you. It looks great, but I am good!" I remind myself that I will feel less energetic after I eat the food being offered, and this usually does it for me. I am making a choice. Occasionally when I run into a food pusher, I say with a smile, "I feel better when I skip _____." I am thankful someone is offering me something they enjoy, but this doesn't mean it works for me. I teach my clients to do the same thing. If this is a hard concept for you, rehearse it in your own words. You are the only one who will have to live with the long-term consequences. If someone has an issue with you making healthier choices, it is his or her issue, not yours. Say a prayer for them and change the subject.

Do You Eat to Relax or Do You Relax When You Eat?

Along with entertaining and being entertained comes relaxation. You need to relax. It is also easier to be temperate when you are relaxed. However, using food to relax doesn't work because trying to use food for something for which it was not intended leads to overeating. Instead, take a deep breath and pray before you eat. This simple act helps you to relax. It puts God in between you and whatever you are stressed out about. It also puts God in between you and food. Processed food and alcohol are not stress reducers. God is. In many cases, processed foods create stress. When you eat junk, you are just adding another stressor because junk is hard work for your body to process. You are not refueling or helping yourself heal from the day's bombardments. Instead, you are contributing to your stress. The truth hurts, but this is a key concept to understand.

Finally, sit down to eat. Many seem to think if they stand while eating, those calories don't count. The other problem you may have when standing is that you may never really feel satisfied since you are in a grazing mode. Even if it is the perfect grass-fed, organic, free-range meal, standing up and wolfing it down all stressed out doesn't pair well with digestion. Without a beginning or an end to a meal, people seem to keep eating. Sitting at the beginning and standing at the end seems to cue a start and a finish.

To Carb or Not to Carb

There is so much confusion over carbohydrates these days. The FAITH VS. WEIGHT philosophy is that your total carbohydrate intake should be linked to your activity level. Although many consider walking to the car their workout, most people take in enough carbs to fuel a daily ultramarathon. Although the type of carb, amount, and timing are hotly debated, carbs are not bad. At least everyone agrees on vegetables. So, there we have consensus. However, depending on the amount of carbs allowed in a specific diet, even types of vegetables are contested. Below is an explanation of diets with different carbohydrate options, including the FAITH VS. WEIGHT Diet plan.

Ketogenic Diets

Ketogenic diets (extremely low carb) stick with non-starchy vegetables as the carbohydrate of choice, with very limited fruit, if any. These diets are high in fat and moderate in protein. If you want wow results, ketogenic is the way to go. However, most ketogenic diets are only recommended for a period of time. I don't see many women thriving on ultra-low carb as a permanent solution. I believe this is because premenopausal women have higher carbohydrate needs than men. As for postmenopausal, it seems to be a case-by-case basis. (There are medically supervised ketogenic diets used for specific health reasons beyond weight management.)

Low-Carb Diets

Low-carb diets are less stringent than ketogenic and may allow some starchy vegetables and fruits. These diets tend to be moderate in protein and fat. Low carb has significant benefits over the standard American diet (SAD), but it is also difficult for many to stick with over the long haul. Unfortunately, I see many who have gained weight after rebounding from low-carb diets. However, there is a thing or two to be learned from low carb. The benefits of a low-carb diet are its convenience and ability to help eliminate sugar cravings. Many lose weight on low-carb diets. You may also notice that your energy is higher after a low-carb meal versus a higher-carb meal. However, over time you may run out of gas or have trouble sleeping, as I did.

Moderate Carb Diets

Moderate carb eating allows for non-starchy and starchy carb vegetables, fruits, legumes, and grains. The FAITH VS. WEIGHT Diet is a moderate carb diet with a twist. On the FVW plan, the carbs for breakfast, lunch, and snacks are limited to fifteen to twenty grams and are composed primarily of vegetables with some low-glycemic fruit. Starchy carbs like grains and tubers are enjoyed at night. Vegetables (starchy and non-starchy) are enjoyed at lunch, while low-glycemic fruits at breakfast and for snacks keep both energy levels and fat burning high. During the day, you will eat the right type and amount of carbs to fuel energy requirements without excess to store as fat (See eating timing and tips chart.) As your body needs more energy, it will use your stored fat. At dinner or after dinner, starchy carbohydrates (grains, potatoes) are introduced in order to prepare for sleep. When eaten within a short time of having protein, which contains tryptophan, carbohydrates trigger serotonin production, a good friend of a good night's sleep.

Carbohydrate intake should be tied to your activity level. You will find less active and more active options on the eating timing and tips chart. Less active clients enjoy a starchy carbohydrate and dessert and then stop eating after dinner. If you are in the more active category, you may want an after-dinner snack. Everyone has the same hundred-calorie option for dessert. On this plan, more active does not mean more dessert. However, it may mean more starchy carbohydrates. All options are listed on the eating timing and tips chart. Find your starchy carb sweet spot. You will know based on how well you sleep and how hungry you are the next day if you had enough to eat the previous night. The eating timing and tips chart shows an after-dinner snack of one hundred calories of starchy carbohydrate plus one hundred calories of plant based fat. If you are very active, you can increase your starchy carbohydrate intake to two hundred calories.

Sleep Please!

Most who try the FAITH VS. WEIGHT Diet plan are shocked with how much more energy they have during the day. After avoiding starchy carbs earlier in the day and feeling better, some wonder … why not skip starchy carbs all together? This would put you in the low-carb category. Instead, if you follow this plan, you will maintain the convenience and increased energy of the lower end of a moderate carb-eating plan during the day with the added benefit of higher starchy carbs at night cueing the body for sleep. This means you will have more energy for the next day. Once I switched from having oatmeal for breakfast to having it at night, I felt more energetic in the mornings and slept better at night. Most people don't realize how starchy carbs affect their morning energy until they skip them in the mornings. The breakfasts on this plan will leave you feeling alert. Clients report better energy during the day with deeper sleep at night on the FAITH VS. WEIGHT diet plan. Another sleep trick is to stop drinking water after dinner. The eating timing and tips chart outlines when to hydrate. This results in almost zero middle-of-the-night bathroom trips.

TIMING IS EVERYTHING

With The FAITH VS. WEIGHT diet, you have the option to eat starchy carbohydrates at dinner, after dinner, or split between both, depending on your activity level. All combinations are listed in the appendix lunch/dinner and eating timing and tips charts. The appendix also has a restaurant plan showing the "at dinner" carbohydrate recommendations if you want to have a starchy carb at dinner at a restaurant. If you are in the more active category and want to skip carbs at dinner, you can still have a small dessert, sticking with protein, extra vegetables, and plant-based fats at restaurants, while later having your starchy carb option as an after-dinner snack. All combinations are listed. If you are less active and want to skip the starchy carb at a restaurant, you can always have a hundred calories of popcorn when you get home as part of your dinner.

The reason to consider skipping starchy carbs at restaurants is because they rarely have healthy options, and the portions are gargantuan. If you only eat at restaurants that have the healthy starchy carbs listed on the lunch/dinner chart, you will be very limited. If you decide to have a hundred-calorie popcorn snack when you get home, you can eat at practically any restaurant and not worry about the quality of a restaurant's starchy carbs. You also won't have to worry about overdoing it. At almost any restaurant, you can find a protein, vegetable, and fat, and last time I checked, they all still have dessert. Enjoy a decaf coffee or herbal tea and keep your dessert to a hundred calories. A ballpark estimate is no more than a quarter cup. Sipping a hot herbal tea or decaf coffee and savoring your dessert makes it last longer. You can always go home later and enjoy your hundred calories of popcorn or oatmeal. No deprivation here!

Not only have starchy carbs at night improved my client's sleep, their percent of body fat also decreased. Since total carb intake is more of an issue than time of day, you might as well eat an appropriate amount of starchy carbs at night when they are less likely to decrease morning energy levels, triggering sugar cravings, and more likely to help you sleep. If you follow this plan and limit your starchy carbs to either dinner, after dinner, or split between both as described in the lunch/dinner chart, you will discover you can lose weight while eating carbs at night. When you are already very active and eating healthy, the scale may not move much one way or the other, but that doesn't mean you are not losing fat. Your clothes will tell you.

The distribution and type of carbs on this plan have given my clients their greatest energy gains along with their greatest sustainable weight loss success without feeling deprived. You still may be thinking if this is all about total carbs, then why not have starchy carbs earlier in the day, especially if starchy carbs don't make you feel sleepy during the day. Just like sugar, starchy carbohydrates earlier in the day tend to cause cravings for more starchy car-bohydrates and sugar the rest of the day. This is another reason why starchy carbs and dessert are at night on this plan. Alertness was also higher for my clients during the day when they had starchy carbs at night. If you have not already, take a picture of the first three charts of the appendix and try it for three days. It is much easier to be temperate when cravings are in check and you are eating at regular intervals. Another reason to have starchy carbs after dinner instead of at dinner is because this allows you to be able to go *anywhere* for dinner and enjoy a protein with non-starchy veggies and fat. You don't have to worry about finding decent carbs at restaurants. It is much easier at home to have your high-quality starchy carb after dinner, giving you a good night's sleep and energy for the next day's workout. This sets you up to be more temperate in your choices tomorrow, not just today.

Skip the Gluten

Finally, the biggest caution other than type, amount, and timing of carbohydrates is gluten. There is just no upside to gluten. However, gluten-free, especially in processed products, doesn't necessarily mean weight loss friendly because these products can spike blood sugar even higher than the carbs they replace. Many starches are naturally gluten-free and are also listed on the lunch/dinner chart. Oats can be exposed to gluten if they are not prepared in a gluten-free facility. The steel cut oatmeal I eat for my after-dinner snack is gluten-free because it is cut in a gluten-free facility. If oatmeal is gluten-free, it is labeled as gluten-free.

Dessert or No Dessert

When you are at a restaurant and make good food choices (lean protein, some healthy fat, and lots of veggies with an optional sprinkle of cheese) and you want to partake in a shared dessert, choose a small amount to put on a separate plate and savor it slowly. The community trough is not your weight loss friend. Putting a small amount on a separate plate is a visual cue. Instead, if you keep digging into the community trough, you will have no idea how much you have eaten and no cue as to when to stop. Three small bites on a small plate, known as the "the three-bite rule," savored over time provides the maximum satisfaction with the minimal damage. We are going to guesstimate this as one hundred calories since there is no label on restaurant desserts. Beyond that, you encounter the law of diminishing returns. More is not better when it comes to sugar or your waistline.

If the hundred calories suggested for dessert on the FAITH VS. WEIGHT diet seems inadequate, let's do the math. Per week: 7 x 100 = 700 calories; per year: 52 x 700 = 36,400 calories. This number does not include up to three glasses of wine a week, which is currently the max suggested for breast cancer prevention. If you drink up to three glasses of only four ounces of wine per week (which is less than what is served in restaurants), you are adding 60,000 calories a year in the form of sugar or fermented sugar. Do you really need more sugar?

If it is too hard to be temperate with restaurant desserts, substitutions are available on the FAITH VS. WEIGHT diet. Some clients prefer nuts, pop-corn, or 70 percent or greater dark chocolate. Others prefer dark chocolate in higher percentages than 70 percent since the higher the percentage of cacao, the less sugar to cause cravings.

> For God is not a God of disorder but of peace.
>
> —1 Corinthians 14:33 (NIV)

Temperance does not necessarily mean avoiding something altogether. However, it does mean not overdoing it. Temperance is the peaceful balance of having your house in order. Balance means not overdoing or underdoing it, which causes chaos for your mind and body, whether it is with food or alcohol. Do you often over or underdo it because the devil convinces you that you can't win, so why bother? If there is something repeatedly causing you to go into chaos mode, distracting you from God's call on your life, consider this your wake-up call to ask for help in overcoming it. For some it is sugar, and for others it is something else. "I just want to get control of my eating" are often the first words new clients say to me. They feel like their eating is controlling them. Sadly, they are right. I know because I have been there. You are not alone!

In the previous chapter, we discussed how practicing prudence begs the question, "What is the most likely outcome of what I am about to do?" The reason prudence comes before temperance is because you may not be able to be temperate in all things. For example, if you are an alcoholic, you are probably not going to be temperate with alcohol. So in order to practice self-control, it would be prudent to skip it all together. This is where an all-or-nothing mentality can actually save your life. In my early years as a navy officer, I developed a navy drug and alcohol rehab tracking program. I was immensely blessed to see firsthand significant numbers of people putting their lives back together after rehabbing from drugs and alcohol. One of the most highly respected professionals I worked with was a recovering alcoholic who had over twenty years of sobriety. Every day at lunch, he read his Bible. I would bet that was not the only time. He was an inspiration to all.

THIN MINTS, ANYONE?

Recovering alcoholics know they cannot be temperate with alcohol. The same goes with certain people with certain foods. If someone struggling for years with an alcohol addiction can save their life by changing their habits, you can conquer your battle with food. If you have a certain food you cannot be temperate with at this time, it would be prudent for you to avoid it. Get the idea? Years ago, when the Girl Scouts knocked on my door selling Thin Mints, I gave them a donation. I did not buy any cookies because I used to go through a sleeve of Thin Mints in one day! I decided to be prudent and not bring them into the house. Following the FAITH VS. WEIGHT diet plan, I was able to reintroduce Thin Mints and be happy with two cookies a day for dessert. I would buy the cookies, have my two after my FAITH VS. WEIGHT dinner, and be done with it. I had learned how to be temperate, which is exactly what you will learn as you follow this program.

Most of my clients continue to have their dessert every day as described on this plan and lose weight. This plan has helped them become temperate, as I was with my two Thin Mint cookies. Whatever you prefer, once you are temperate with a food category, you can make a decision as to whether or not you want to take it or leave it. This is the opposite of what most people do every day with sugar. The majority of people seesaw between having tons of sugar to no sugar, binging or denying as they continue to go back and forth with an all-or-nothing mentality. This does not work. If there is a particular food or drink causing chaos, you are better off acknowledging it by being prudent and avoiding it. However, unnecessary deprivation is not required in order to be temperate and usually backfires. Most people are not ready to give up the entire category of dessert, just because certain desserts trigger a binge. Finding what works for you is worth the effort. The only way to do this is to follow the plan and cut down on sugar during the day so that you can actually figure out what works as a dessert; otherwise you will remain enslaved in a state of chaos.

A sustained effort to reduce your sugar intake will allow you to make the decision instead of sugar making the decision for you. Again, if you never get to this decision point with a particular food, it may belong in the prudence category. Different foods trigger different things in different people. The higher the sugar content, the harder it is to have just one: think candy corns. This is why I recommend 70 percent or higher dark chocolate for people who want to spend a hundred calories on a dessert. I also often recommend Alter Eco black truffles. These are not quite at 70 percent, but they contain a small amount of coconut oil, which is highly satiating. Salt is another trigger. Think of the classic example of salted versus unsalted nuts. This also applies to dark chocolate with sea salt. Salted desserts encourage more eating. You are better off with unsalted.

It is always easier to be temperate with real food. Nowadays, the term "food" is a misnomer for processed food products, since most of these are a cocktail of chemicals. No wonder many of us are fat and have constant cravings. There is no way of knowing which of the hundreds of chemicals are triggering your cravings. We are an "overfed and undernourished nation." This is a popular concept being conveyed to create awareness as to what we are eating. In the beginning, to build your confidence, get rid of whatever you are unable to be temperate with until you can be temperate in all things you are currently consuming. This will build confidence. Eating real food is the only place to start.

Eating a sleeve of Thin Mints daily bothered me more than the extra weight. Along with robbing my confidence, I knew I was not being temperate. I did not have a name for it then, but the Holy Spirit convicted me nonetheless. Most people are not just unhappy because they have extra weight; they are unhappy because of their behavior. This is an area where we need a little or a lot of help. This is not about guilt. This is about awareness. Once you are aware of your triggers, you will feel less helpless and can make prudent decisions that lead to an overall temperate diet.

Make Your Move

Because the foolishness of God is wiser than men, and the weakness of
God is stronger than men.

—*1 Corinthians 1:25 (WEB)*

We also seem to lack temperance when it comes to exercise. We are either doing too much or too little. There are a lot of misperceptions surrounding exercise and caloric intake when it comes to weight loss. Licensing is a psychological behavior that feeds these erroneous beliefs. The thought process goes along these lines, "Because I did *x*, now I deserve *y*." Because I had a killer workout, now I deserve a pint of ice cream. It's also more commonly misapplied to stress. Since I had a miserable day at work, I deserve the nachos supreme at happy hour in lieu of my workout. Instead, try turning to exercise as a stress reducer. Although stress starts in your head based on how you react to things, you feel the tension in your body. Trying to sedate it only makes things worse. You are better off unleashing it. Exercise is a great answer for stress for a multitude of reasons, but one of the most overlooked reasons is it releases physical tension. Gross motor exercise such as walking stimulates the parasympathetic nervous system, which helps you relax. Something as simple as going for a walk right after work is a great way to relieve stress, also minimizing the opportunity to overeat!

As much as exercise is underestimated as a stress reducer, it is overestimated as a weight-loss tool. The truth is exercise lies somewhere in the middle. A killer workout does not mean you earned the right to eat a thousand calories in one sitting. You may think the more painful your workout, the higher the caloric burn. This is another weight-loss myth. Even if this were true, if something is too hard, you will not be able to sustain it. How painful your workout is has nothing to do with how many calories you've burned. Weekend warriors wind up with more injuries than weight loss. I see many people at the gym going for killer workouts, thinking they are now able to eat whatever they want because they are sore. On top of that, they tend to be inactive the rest of the day, which actually leads to weight gain and heart disease.

Another misperception when it comes to caloric intake is "If I feel like I am starving, then I must be losing weight." Not eating enough can slow your metabolism. This results in your body storing every calorie. Starving yourself is also a surefire way to set yourself up for a trip through the nearest drive-through, and you are most probably not going to order the salad. If you are not doing any cardio, find a twenty-minute window and start moving. Getting your day started on the right foot by listening to worship music or an audio version of the Bible is practicing preventative stress management. After work is another ideal time to release stress, but almost any time is a good time for exercise. Many cultures around the world go for a walk after dinner to digest their food. If this is not practical, pick a time of day during a lunch break and listen to an audio book or music while you go for a walk or climb stairs. If you are outside, pay attention to your surroundings. Plan on some type of movement every day. I find that clients who plan on exercising five days wind up doing three. If you plan on doing it three days, it may only happen on one. It is actually easier to stick with exercise when it is a daily rather than sporadic commitment. If you do something daily, it is more likely to become a habit. I don't recommend doing the same type or intensity of exercise every day, but I do recommend moving daily. If you do some form of exercise on most days, your body will tend to expect it, and you will be more likely to find ways to make it happen.

Before Bed

Eat according to the plan based on your activity level. Many new clients tell me they overeat at night because they are bored, lonely, tired, wired, and so on. Occasionally you may also overdo it because you have not eaten enough during the day, and now you are starving. Whatever the case, eating accord-ing to the plan will help keep your energy levels steady, which will help you to not overdo it at night. Evening is the time to start winding down. Do not abuse your digestive system, making it work harder keeping your body up half of the night trying to digest whatever junk was available. Think "soothing" and "comfort" instead of more food. Do evening stretches to prepare for sleep or take a hot shower or enjoy a warm bath to release tension and induce calm.

Take a Stand

REBELLION: WHO'S IN CHARGE HERE?

Many new clients confide, "My boss (my kids, my husband, my ex, etc.) was making me crazy, so I wound up overdoing it." It's human nature to have conflict. In some cases, a third party is needed like a counselor (love counselors!) to sort things out. But I am pretty sure when it comes to what we put in our mouths, I have yet to see anyone putting a gun to our head, forcing us to polish off a sleeve of Thin Mints (maybe this was just my excuse). Just because someone is acting awful does not mean you should beat yourself up in the process. I have even heard so-and-so make snotty comments, or maybe they were meant to be "helpful" (if translated in another language), about your progress or "lack of it" when you were trying to make healthy lifestyle improvements. Super. There is only one problem. So-and-so is not going to take or pay for your diabetes meds or drive you to chemo.

MIND YOUR TEMPER

What is the root word of temperance? Temper is not just associated with losing it. Temper is also about balance. If you lose your temper because you are angry, you are off balance. Many people are angry with themselves for a variety of reasons, including weight gain. These are usually the same people who get the most easily angered with others. Clients often tell me they are angry with themselves for gaining weight. I explain to them weight gain happens a lot faster than people realize, which is the reason to pay attention moving forward. Ask for help in forgiving yourself. Since the Lord has already forgiven you, it is vain for you not to forgive yourself. Anger will keep you fat. In order to forgive others, you have to forgive yourself first. One day you will be judged in the same way you judge others, so that is a good reason to forgive anyone who has wronged you, starting now, including yourself! Then let it go. Sometimes it's actually good to have a bad memory!

> Brothers, I don't regard myself as yet having taken hold, but one thing I do. Forgetting the things which are behind, and stretching forward to the things which are before.
>
> —Philippians 3:13 (WEB)

Many clients also initially rebel against the person they are paying for and asking advice from. It is human nature to want to be in charge, but if you are fighting the person who is trying to help you, are you really interested in being helped in the first place? As my husband loves to remind me, "You can't listen when you are talking." This is my cue to shut it and start learning from whoever I have just asked or hired to help me, instead of resisting, questioning, and doubting their help the entire time. Humility is the best teacher. Ask yourself, "Who exactly are you rebelling against?" Use your energy to become better instead of bitter and allow yourself some grace. No one requires you to learn a new job in one day, so give yourself the same latitude in changing lifelong behaviors. This next chart gives you three simple steps to help you ease into it.

FAITH VS. WEIGHT Process

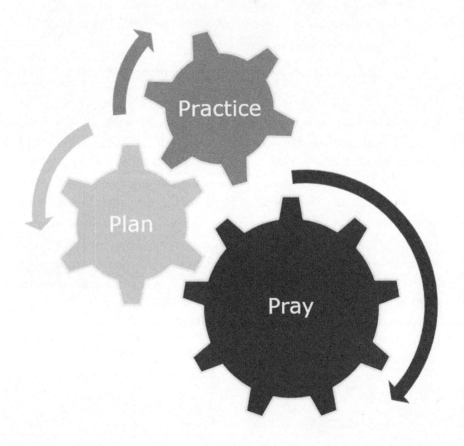

In the beginning, you may have a 50 percent success rate. The more times you engage in this process, the better your results will be. Try a goal of 80 percent plus for success!

Pray

Instead of wasting your energy being angry at yourself or someone else when you overdo it, pray to forgive yourself and others. Ask for guidance to do better next time.

Practice

Like I tell my kids, "What is the difference between hard and easy? Practice!" Rewind your mind and practice a better outcome next time. Visualization is a powerful tool used by Olympic athletes.

Plan

Planning can mean the difference between forty to fifty pounds of weight loss per year. Did you forget your afternoon snack before you went to the dinner party starving? Sometimes it's an obvious fix, but you still have to plan for a better outcome in order to avoid a repeat performance.

Love Your Neighbor

Self-Discipline = Self-Respect = Self-Love

As a believer in the Lord Jesus Christ, you already have all of the self-discipline you will ever need to do whatever it is He is calling you to do. God does not call you to do something without equipping you to do it. However, you still have to answer the call.

One of my roommates in my early Navy days used to jot down the above saying when she would doodle. I am not sure of the exact order since it was thirty years ago, but these were the words. This motto helped her to fulfill her calling to serve as a Marine Corps Officer. She had a very successful career, but first went through Boot Camp, and then an Officer Training Prep Program before eventually earning an NROTC Scholarship, which led to her commission as a Marine Corps Officer. This was a long process, and it would have been easier to give up than to pursue. I know how hard it was. Although I was commissioned as a Navy Officer, our first four years of training were similar. Her doodling kept me going when I wanted to quit.

Fulfilling your calling inspires others to fulfill theirs. In your case, loving yourself enough in order to pursue a healthy lifestyle will inspire others to achieve theirs. Since Jesus wants you to love your neighbor as much as you love yourself, you need to love yourself. There are a lot of people who need to know the love of Christ, and you or I may be their only glimpse at it. Loving yourself enough to pursue your calling to a healthier lifestyle is one way to inspire others to do the same resulting in more energy to serve the kingdom.

CHANGE YOUR LIFE

WEEK TWO: TEMPERANCE

For God didn't give us a spirit of fear, but of power, love, and self-control.

—*2 Timothy 1:7 (WEB)*

FOR YOUR SOUL

Are you focused on God's power or your limitations?

If your why does not seem like a prize worth fighting for, go back to the Bible. Ask Jesus to help you get excited about the why He has planted in your heart.

Is your entitlement mentality keeping you fat? Do you deserve sugar?

Are you an all-or-nothing person? Temperance is a sustained, manageable effort, not a knee-jerk reaction. Ask for peace in order to achieve balance.

What is one habit you can ask for help in changing for the better?

Are you looking for love in all of the wrong places? Addiction is the opposite of temperance. If you look away from God, you will always be looking. Get help if you need it.

Help someone less fortunate than you to feel at home, especially over the holidays. Instead of making it the "eating season," remember the "reason for the season." Choose to worship. Listen/sing Christian Christmas carols.

Forgive as you would like to be forgiven. Start by forgiving yourself.

Write in your NLG (nightly letter to God) asking Him to help you forgive if you are unable to forgive on your own. If you are sincere, He will help you do it.

Pray, practice, plan, repeat.

For Your Body

Ask yourself, "What has food done for me lately?"

Real food allows you to be temperate. Fake food never satisfies.

Remember, this is not the Last Supper.

Special occasion or not? Celebrate instead of wondering why you overate again.

Check out the restaurant guide and restaurant options in the appendix before you dine.

At restaurants:

Start with water and order a veggie appetizer/salad.

Try some tea or decaf coffee with dessert in order to slow down.

Avoid the community trough when it comes to dessert or any shared dish. Ask for a small plate and take an amount no more than a one-fourth cup of dessert. After three bites, it's the law of diminishing returns.

Stick with the eating timing and tips chart on vacation and at home.

Start incorporating regular aerobic exercise for a minimum of twenty minutes a day, shooting for most days of the week. This way you have some wiggle room. Continue to get up and move around within fifteen to twenty minutes after eating. Your twenty minutes of aerobic exercise can count as one of these sessions. Give it your (PB) personal best, not your neighbor's.

WEEK THREE

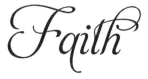

He said to her, "Daughter, your faith has healed you."

—Mark 5:34 (NIV)

He was amazed at their lack of faith.

—Mark 6:6 (NIV)

Your life is not a foregone conclusion. Did you know that every single lifestyle decision you make is affected by your faith or lack of it? When you err on the side of doubt, either consciously or by default, you are not only limiting yourself but also limiting God. Instead, when you choose faith and act on it, you are open to the unlimited power of the Almighty Lord Jesus Christ. Anything can happen. This applies to all areas, including your health and your weight. The reason we don't choose faith in this area is we are afraid of being let down. Doubt, which is basically a lack of faith, almost always has a fear component. The only way to get over this fear is to grow in your faith and then act on it. This chapter is designed to help you to develop a faith that takes action. Why is an active faith so important? Your faith, or lack of it, affects your actions today, which in turn affects your health tomorrow.

According to the Bible, your faith affects your actions, but it can also affect God's actions on your behalf. The Bible dramatically describes different outcomes solely dependent on a person's faith or lack of it. The following verse describes a woman who was suffering for years from a debilitating disease but was healed because of her faith.

> *He said to her, "Daughter, your faith has healed you."*
>
> *—Mark 5:34 (NIV)*

The very next chapter of Mark describes an incident where Jesus's ability to heal and perform miracles was wasted solely because of a lack of faith.

> *He was amazed by their lack of faith.*
>
> *—Mark 6:6 (NIV)*

In the first case, Jesus tells us it was the woman's faith that healed her. He does not take credit for healing her even though her healing came through Him. So if He is not taking the credit and she could not heal herself without Him, how exactly did her faith heal her?

> *Immediately Jesus, perceiving in himself that the power had gone out from him, turned around in the crowd, and asked, "Who touched my clothes?"*
>
> *—Mark 5:30 (WEB)*

He is clearly telling us that when she touched him, "the power had gone out of him." Anybody could have touched His clothes, but only one woman did it in faith. Because of the sheer volume of people, the disciples thought it was ridiculous that Jesus was trying to figure out who touched Him.

> *His disciples said to him, "You see the multitude pressing against you, and you say, "Who touched me?"*
>
> *—Mark 5:31 (WEB)*

Apparently Jesus was not satisfied by this comment …

> *But Jesus kept looking around to see who had done it. Then the woman, knowing what had happened to her, came and fell at his feet and, trembling with fear, told him the whole truth.*
>
> *—Mark 5:32–33 (NIV)*

He wanted everyone, including us, to hear "the whole truth." I imagine she had to share the depth of her despair along with how she believed Jesus was the only one capable of healing her. Apparently she was right. Jesus then told her in front of everyone she was healed because of her faith. He did not say she was healed because she touched Him. He said she was healed because of her faith. That's because Jesus knew she would never have touched Him if it were not for her faith. Her faith had to precede her actions.

First she had to have faith in the power of Jesus in order to access it, and then she had to act on her faith. Without an active faith, she would not have gotten her miracle. If she did not believe Jesus was capable of healing her, she would not have pushed through the crowd. She would not have gotten within an arm's length of His body. She would not have touched his garment. She would not have been healed. None of this would have happened had she not had faith in His ability to heal her and then acted on it. This woman, who had been bleeding for several years, was probably worn out before she even started. Yet her faith was so strong she acted on it.

On Miracles

When it comes to miracles cited in the Bible, we do not always know who had faith and who did not, but in these two cases, there was no question. There are certainly cases where faith may have had nothing to do with why a miracle was performed. Of course there are also cases where people have had great faith, and yet their miracle did not seem to come, at least not according to our timeline or standards. So what do we know about miracles? In all cases, miracles are performed to show God's glory, and when a miracle does occur, the result is either someone coming to faith or strengthening the faith they already have. One way or another, miracles are tied to faith. If you want to be part of a miracle, you can greatly enhance your odds of participation by acting out in faith.

> If you have faith as small as a mustard seed, you can say to this mountain, "Move from here to there," and it will move. Nothing will be impossible for you.
>
> —Matthew 17:20 (NIV)

He can take your mustard seed of faith, the little bit of faith you have right now when it comes to your health, and turn it into something really great if you act on it. When it comes to your health and weight management, are you taking actions that show you have faith in God? If you substituted the woman's condition in the previous passage for your excess weight, would your faith touch Jesus? The woman who was miraculously healed from a condition causing her to bleed for twelve years had spent all her money and been seen by many doctors. Instead of getting better, she just got worse. It would have been easier for her to give up than to have faith. There are many people who feel this way about their weight. Although the situations may differ, the feeling of hopelessness is the same. Imagine what this woman would have let slip through her fingers had she not put her hope in Jesus, had she not acted out in faith?

I know a lot of people who believe they have faith but do not act on it when it comes to their health. Action is a part of faith. What if the woman mentioned above had started thinking it was too hard to get to Jesus or maybe He really couldn't do what she thought He could do? Why wasn't she healed already? Why should she have to push through a crowd to get to Him? What if she was just too tired? Who could blame her? No one. Yet what would she have abandoned had she not acted out in faith in this particular area or at all? Imagine what you may be abandoning by your not acting out in faith.

> He could not do any miracles there, except lay his hands on a few sick people and heal them.
>
> —Mark 6:5 (NIV)

We don't hear much about the miracles Jesus did not perform, but here is a clear example of what happens when faith is lacking. In Mark, chapter 6, not only did the Nazarenes hear about Jesus, they knew Him very well. They happened to be his relatives and childhood friends growing up. Yet they couldn't get past the idea that the person they had known since birth had anything special to offer. Can you imagine being so close to your miracle and not having enough faith to receive it? Of course you can; we do it every day. There are many Christians who have known Jesus since their childhood but do not step out in faith when it comes to this area. Are you one of them? Is it time to take a faith inventory concerning your health? What are your foregone conclusions when it comes to your weight? Do you believe with your whole heart He is more than capable of healing you? If so, then your next step is to step out in faith.

Just as the woman above had to first believe, she then had to act on her belief. In her case, this meant fighting the crowd. In yours, it may mean fighting doubt. It may mean going to the supermarket and buying healthy food again. Maybe it means buying an exercise bike or joining a gym if you haven't already. It will mean picking the menu item with the best nutritional profile. It will mean hydrating and packing your snacks. More importantly, it will mean taking the time to start each new day reading your Bible. Do you want to be in the faith category of the healed woman or of the Nazarenes, assuming it wasn't going to happen anyway, so why bother? The point is this woman had a faith that called her to act. What about you?

DELAYED MIRACLES

There is no one like the God of Jeshurun, who rides across the heavens to help you and on the clouds in his majesty.

—Deuteronomy 33:26 (NIV)

This emphatic statement of praise is what came out of Moses's mouth right after being told by God that he would not be permitted to enter the Promised Land and—oh, by the way—he was going to die. After serving God's people for forty years, Moses pleaded with God to change His mind, but God said no. We have all prayed for a miracle that seemed to never come. We must be in good company since Moses did the same thing. Yet, instead of losing all hope, Moses gave hope. How could he have hope in a God that denied him his miracle after seeing Him perform one miracle after another for the Israelites? He knew firsthand there was no one like this God. Moses gave hope because he had hope in the God of miracles.

No Is an Answer Too

You might assume that if you do not get what you pray for, it must mean you do not have enough faith. Although Moses had his moments of doubt in the past, just like the rest of us, I don't think anyone can accuse him of not having enough faith with this particular request. Yet God still said no. In Deuteronomy 34:10, the Bible says there was not another prophet like Moses whom God knew face-to-face. Even though God said no to this miracle, Moses knew this did not change the fact that God was still the God of miracles. I guess the Lord liked that. In the New Testament, we are told that God didn't just give Moses a glimpse into the Promised Land, the Lord put Moses next to the Messiah, the Lord Jesus Christ, on Mount Tabor. This was a future Moses could not have ever imagined, a future beyond his ability to even comprehend. This was even better than the miracle Moses had hoped and asked for. Maybe, sometimes the Lord has a better miracle in mind.

> *O Lord God, you have only begun to show your servant your greatness and your might; what God in heaven or on earth can perform deeds and mighty acts like yours!*
>
> *—Deuteronomy 3:24 (NRSV)*

Have you given up on believing in miracles because you have been denied? Even though Moses was denied, he still believed in the God of miracles. The Bible gives us many examples of life-changing miracles that occurred while people had plenty of years left on earth. Such examples give us hope in our daily and future struggles. However, just because it doesn't happen on your timeline doesn't mean it's not going to happen. It might even be better than what you asked for.

That is what the Scriptures mean when they say, "No eye has seen, no ear has heard, and no mind has imagined what God has prepared for those who love him."

—*1 Corinthians 2:9 (NLT)*

Love the Lord Your God

So faith comes by hearing, and hearing by the word of God.

—Romans 10:17 (WEB)

Fortunately faith, in all areas, even the ones you have given up on, is not as hard to come by as you might you think. The reason many struggle with faith is that they try to do it on their own. Faith is not a one-person show. Hearing requires two people. We need a speaker and a listener. This is why you were created to be in fellowship with God and other believers. When it comes to your relationship with God, you need to go to the Word of God. One-on-one devotion with Him is often when He speaks to you directly. However, this is not the only source of faith. We are created to be in fellowship with other believers. Find a place of worship where the Word of God is preached. Both time alone with God as well as time with other believers are necessary in order to build your faith muscles.

If you struggle with reading the Bible on a regular basis, you are not alone. Many of my first-time clients go to church and participate in fellowship serving the community but struggle to make daily Bible reading a reality. People have good intentions in this area that never seem to come to fruition. I had tried to read the Bible many times in my life, but I could only handle a passage or two here and there. After checking out the You Version Bible app, I started listening and reading at the same time. Since I realized I couldn't pronounce half of the names in the Bible, listening quickly solved this problem. I also realized I could tell if someone in the Bible was happy, surprised, sarcastic, or mad by listening to the reader's voice inflections. Listening to the Bible is when the Bible came alive for me. In my case, faith really did come from hearing!

I knew that if I didn't commit to a regular time, this was not going to happen on a regular basis. For me, this meant first thing in the morning. Yes, the first mornings were hard, but then my body began waking up before my alarm. By the third day, it was a new habit. I have since cut out some unnecessary nonsense from my day so I can get to sleep when I need to in order to wake up earlier. Since I also exercise in the morning, sometimes I find a way to combine the two. When I travel, you will see me on an exercise bike or treadmill at the gym listening to the Bible. I also do this at home when I do indoor workouts. Instead of binge watching a series late at night, you can spend time with God in the morning, increasing your faith while improving your health! A great way to start your day!

WISDOM IS POWER

In many cases, Christians who consistently read the Bible, applying God's wisdom to everything from their finances and relationships to raising their children, witness to the power of God manifest in their lives. I am one of them! However, when it comes to weight management, wisdom may elude you. We may quote, "Your body is a temple of the Holy Spirit ... You are not your own" —1 Corinthians 6:19 (WEB), but that is the extent of it. Even when your weight-loss efforts start off well, over the long haul, they may dwindle. It only takes one selfie at a bad angle or one iffy comment from a family member and you start doubting. Others have lost faith in this area before they even got started. Some days, you may feel as if you are more likely to get struck by lightning than lose the weight and keep it off. What we lack is patience. If you are willing to be patient enough to seek God's wisdom to get a college degree, save money to buy your first home, advance in your career, and help your child with learning difficulties, weight loss should be no exception. Each requires patience and a daily commitment. We may not go to the first college of our choice or start off with our dream job, but we still take classes and show up at work. In the meantime, we trust God's plan. Faith is not counting on your knowledge of what you consider the perfect fit. Faith is counting on God's wisdom to put you where you belong. In the case of weight management, faith is not counting on a specific number on the scale. Faith is applying the power of His wisdom to our food and exercise choices. In this case, your numbers may look even better than you could have imagined! I have seen this time and again with my clients.

*Now to him who is able to do exceedingly abundantly above all that
we ask or think, according to the power that works in us.*

—*Ephesians 3:20 (WEB)*

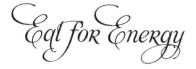

The Two-Year Gym Experiment

Once I was a member of a Jewish Community Center (JCC) in the Bay Area and loved it! However, during my two pregnancies, I wound up suspending my membership as I swam closer to home. About two years later, I returned to the JCC. I might not have noticed the following changes in members' fitness levels had I been there the whole time:

In two years, some of the members remained relatively unchanged.

In two years, some of the members declined in their fitness level.

In two years, a few of the members dramatically improved. They were barely recognizable!

I realized it had been for these people:

Two years of getting in the car and driving in Bay Area traffic to come to the gym

Two years of paying membership fees and dues

Two years of sacrificing family time, free time, work time, and leisure

This scenario is not unique to the JCC. This same scenario plays out in every gym across the country. So how did the few people who were able to achieve it make such amazing progress? Every single one of them cleaned up their diet and added strength and interval training. I couldn't have had a more powerful imprint in my brain of what smart eating and resistance exercise along with interval cardio training can do. Since it had been two years, it was almost like seeing a before-and-after video. It was crystal clear that jogging on the treadmill, while subsisting on processed foods, was not going to cut it. Strength training while eating burgers and fries isn't going to get you there either. If you want results, you need to do both.

You may want to ask yourself, "Have I really worked this hard to get to this stage of life, to make these sacrifices to raise a family, to improve my education, to make partner in my firm, to run a successful company, or to hit a milestone birthday in order to waste my time?" Because this is what most people are doing at the gym. Exercising some is better than none, but exercise has never been proven as an efficient way to lose weight on its own. As my first trainer in the Navy, Petty Officer Harris, used to say, "Fitness doesn't start in the gym." Think of what you could accomplish in three or six months, let alone two years, if you continued to clean up your eating, incorporate strength training, and add interval cardio some to most of the time. Maybe the term "experiment" was a strong word to use for the subtitle of this section. This was not exactly a double-blind clinical control study, but does it matter? The results would still be the same.

Same Circus, Different Clowns

Although the above section sounded like a gym story, it really was an eating story. Only the resistance training and interval cardio part happened in the gym. Interval training, increasing your speed every three to five minutes while doing cardio, is much more efficient than just racking up mileage, causing wear and tear on your knees on the treadmill. Strength training only requires resistance. It does not require heavy loads. However, the main point here is what happens the other twenty-three hours of the day, when not in the gym.

You might be tempted to loosen up a little bit as time goes on. What's the big deal with the 3:00 p.m. stop at your buddy's candy jar on the way to the printer or the second piece of cake for an anniversary, birthday, promotion, or baby shower at work? These were all "special" occasions. Does it make a difference that the healthy salad you ordered in the cafeteria for lunch had the fat and sugar content of an éclair? It's green, right? Besides, the dressing, candied nuts, and cranberries have antioxidants. That's what the package says! Oops! In the real world, cranberries are actually not sweet. And since you had a virtuous salad, surely you are now entitled to the cookies left over in the break room. Besides, you did the elliptical the day before yesterday. You were just going to have one, but somehow you seem to keep finding reasons to make just one more copy and take another pass through. For now, your pants are feeling kind of tight, but aren't things supposed to "shift" as we get older? What difference does it make?

Ask me in two years.

Jesus Doesn't Settle, and Neither Should You!

Why are we settling for this? Settling in one area of your life usually leads to an expectation of mediocrity in others. You were not created to settle. What other area of your life would you spend the same amount of time and money you spend on diet and fitness, settling for lackluster results? You don't have to have an MBA to figure out this is a lousy return on your investment. We almost expect this area to be a net loss. On top of that, we wind up just blaming ourselves. Most people do not give up because they are lazy. They give up because of a lack of faith. Most have lost faith in their ability to make sustained progress with diet and exercise. You are not going to take care of your health if you do not believe you have a chance at attaining your dream of a healthy lifestyle. Have you abandoned this dream? God did not create you to settle. He has a vision for your life and health. It's a big kingdom, and someone has to be His hands and feet. There is plenty of work to be done. You have got to take better care of yourself in order to do it. Since being overweight is now the norm in our society, many don't think they have settled when it comes to taking care of their health. Would you want your kids to feel the same way about their health as most adults do? Is this our new normal? They deserve a healthier vision for their tomorrow.

Unfortunately, just this morning I spoke with an orthopedic nurse who discussed a patient about to undergo a leg amputation due to diabetes. This is an everyday occurrence in our hospitals, with no end in sight. We also have children who are seen every day in the US with diabetes. Is what we are eating worth this? If what we are eating is something we can't live without, then why is it killing us?

It's almost impossible to settle once you are inspired, and it's impossible to be inspired without faith. The two coexist.

Change Your Brain

When I jump to conclusions, my husband reminds me of the difference between correlation and causation. Just because something is associated with something (correlation) does not mean it will automatically cause it (causation). Having rampant obesity in your family does not mean you are doomed to the same fate. When I teach classes, I ask the following questions: "Who do you limit when you believe something is impossible for God?" Everyone points to herself. "Who else do you limit when you believe something is impossible for God?" After thinking about, everyone points to the ceiling. Remember, your life is not a foregone conclusion. You are not the only variable. Isn't that why Jesus came? So you could have new life in Him. When you overcome a struggle in His name, He gets the glory. Oftentimes this is the whole point of struggle. You are delivered, and He is glorified regardless of whatever the struggle is. Just because you've tried countless diets, plans, and gyms doesn't mean you will never see the light at the end of this tunnel. Still, it's worth asking why this program should be any different from the ones you have already tried. You might make assumptions like this one: "If I have failed at every other diet/exercise attempt, this one will be no different." First off, you have not failed; you have succeeded in finding ways that did not work for you.

Regardless of one's personal faith, I see the same look in people's eyes when the topic of losing weight first comes up and again at the midway point. It starts with a flash of hope, then a twinge of fear, and ultimately resignation. It's almost as if they see an oasis in a desert turning out to be quicksand. The warning signs appear, shouting, "Keep out. Don't fall for it! It's a mirage!" This happens in health care facilities multiple times a day when doctors have to tell their patients to lose weight. It's not that we don't want to lose weight; we have just concluded we are too weak to make better choices, and we are correct. This is exactly what Satan wants us to believe. However, the point of this book is not to dwell on the knowledge of our weaknesses but to apply the power of God's wisdom to our choices.

To God belong wisdom and power; counsel and understanding are his.

—Job 12:13 (NIV)

Just as your faith is not a foregone conclusion, neither is your weight. Your weight is simply based on a series of choices made over a period of time. That's it. Once medical issues have been ruled out, anyone who tells you anything else is lying. For most people, it is about choices. The choices you make are influenced by whether or not you want to lose weight, and whether or not you believe you can do it with God's help. If you have already ruled God out of this equation, the devil has won. You will continue to focus on your own weaknesses. Many Bible-believing Christians who have faith in God struggle with weakness in this area. Your weakness is not holding you back. It is your focus on your weakness that is holding you back. Instead, when you focus on God's ability to help you make better choices, you access God's power, just like the woman who was healed by touching Jesus.

He has said to me. "My grace is sufficient for you, for my power is made perfect in weakness." Most gladly therefore I will rather glory in my weaknesses, that the power of Christ may rest on me.

—2 Corinthians 12:9 (WEB)

Lose the Labels

Investing your time and energy in any weight loss program is a leap of faith. You must act in the present moment with an eye on the future. If you are struggling, ask yourself and God what you can do to overcome blaming something or someone else, even if that someone is yourself. If you are still stuck, keep asking. The problem is too many people give up too soon and quit asking. I ask God to reveal things to me every single day, multiple times a day. No one else can give better advice. You have a choice. You can believe in your Creator's ability to help you change your life or you can believe in whatever self-imposed labels you have allowed to stick.

Shallow Waters

The rest of this section deals with assumptions related to yourself or your circumstances that ebb and flow like waves at low tide barely noticeable, except for the undertow that will suck the life out of you if you let it. You may not identify with some of these, but keep an open mind and ask yourself if any of these beliefs about you or your circumstances may be embedded in your brain as a foregone conclusion. Exposing these issues is the first step toward health and fullness of life.

Got Doubt?

> *But let him ask in faith, without any doubting, for he who doubts is like a wave of the sea, driven by the wind and tossed.*
>
> *—James 1:6 (WEB)*

If you are still wondering, "Do you really think I can lose the weight?" you are not alone. This is the number one question either asked or thought by every client. The next question to ask yourself is, "Why not?" Do you think your friend can do it or your neighbor down the street? Do they possess superpowers you do not? There is no reason for people medically cleared not to lose weight when they eat healthy and exercise. Yet doubt is the number one thing most people have to overcome. Although losing weight happens on a meal-by-meal basis, the ultimate reward may seem far off. Instead of obsessing over the scale, start measuring success by your energy level after each meal. If you have been following the plan so far, then you are probably in the category of most of my clients who are amazed they are losing weight, but the first thing I hear is they have more energy. They can tell a big difference in their energy level. Again, instead of obsessing over the scale, start measuring success by your energy level after each meal. This is immediate feedback, and it will build confidence eventually getting you to your goal. In case you are afraid you will not be able to stick with it because of your schedule, this program is meant for people on the go. You will have to do some planning, but the planning required is no more than necessary in any other area of your life. As a matter of fact, it is less, while the energy you gain will improve your chance of success in other areas.

Would you reject your dream job because you have to fill out an application? Once you get the job, don't you have an initial adjustment period? Do you think that today you will do your best, but tomorrow you will slack off? Chances are you wouldn't be in the position very long with that attitude. Don't you have to do some planning to reach your goals in this job? On second thought, maybe it's too hard; maybe you should not apply at all. Besides, you might not even get the job. It sounds too hard.

Although the above may sound like nonsense, it happens more often than not when it comes to dieting. Whatever you do, don't let doubt make decisions for you. There are enough people who will say no to you in your life; don't add to the list by saying no to yourself. If you happen to be in the category where you are struggling to eat healthy with your current schedule, pack food the night before or the morning of. There are also plenty of zero-cook and restaurant options provided. If you are already eating healthy, it may mean just tweaking 100–200 calories a day (usually carbohydrates or fats) over time. Many people think they are eating healthy, but they are still taking in more refined carbohydrates and sugar then they like to admit, even to themselves. You may need more protein. You may need a way to wake up your metabolism with more movement, interval training, or an adjustment to your strength-training routine. Frequency and categories of exercises will be covered in this and upcoming chapters.

LACK CONFIDENCE?

A lack of confidence is different from doubt. Doubt is usually over a specific issue or issues. Lack of confidence is more pervasive. In certain situations, we have a very low tolerance for it. As an information systems officer in the navy, I was first stationed with an aircraft squadron before later working in hospitals. It didn't take long to notice certain similarities among certain professions. Both pilots and surgeons have to make life-and-death decisions under highly stressful situations. People in these fields also tend to be confident in their ability to get the job done. They may not be confident in other areas, but put them in a cockpit or in an OR, and they get the job done. However, pilots are not born flying out of the womb, and as far as I know, there haven't been many toddlers performing surgery. Practice builds confidence. First the steps are learned, and then multiple drills are performed so certain reactions become second nature. Obviously every situation is different, but during training drills, procedures are practiced over and over again so the most likely potential life-and-death case scenarios are averted. Certain default behaviors are established. Once a plan of action is decided on, there is no time to think about each step or question, "Gee, what should I do next?" In these cases, learned behavior is similar to a computer default. Similarly, you make life-or-death decisions every day about your health. Your current state of health can be linked to a series of choices over time. In order to build confidence, you need to practice making healthy decisions over and over again. We've already had plenty of practice making unhealthy ones—so much so we do not even believe we can make healthy ones anymore. This is another lie from the father of lies.

When he speaks a lie, he speaks on his own; for he is a liar.

—John 8:44 (WEB)

The devil does a great job of undermining confidence. Most people are not aware of this, but it is true. Only faith in Jesus Christ is strong enough to overcome lies from the enemy. With His help, you can set new neural pathways and train your brain to make healthy decisions. This may not come easily at first, but it absolutely, without a doubt, can become second nature if you let it. Your goal is for your new default behavior to make the healthiest choices possible. Practice builds habits. Your healthy choices can become second nature. Opportunities to make better food choices exist, whether we want to admit it or not. This may mean bringing your own food or having a snack before an event. You may decide ahead of time you will only eat certain food groups (protein and veggies) at a restaurant or party and bring a hundred calories of nuts along as your healthy fat.

Trust in the Lord with all your heart and lean not on your own understanding.

—Proverbs 3:5 (NIV)

When a client tells me she has fallen off the wagon, I ask her to replay specific unsuccessful events in her mind and rehearse each one with a happier ending. Practicing positive outcomes builds confidence since it increases the likelihood for success! Practice also builds habits. Do not underestimate the power of your habits. I bet if you woke up from a coma, and I gave you certain healthy foods every day for a number of days, and you had no idea of how you ate before the coma, this type of eating would become your new normal!

No Discipline?

The military knows about discipline. Boot camp and officer training give you two options: Option 1: do everything it takes to get through training so you can graduate and serve your country. Option 2: fail to do everything it takes to get through training, and you will repeat it or fail out. Most military induction training periods are not fun experiences no matter what one's natural proclivity is toward discipline, and most people do not want to prolong or repeat these experiences. On top of that, most people do not like to fail. In this case, people from all walks of life are willing to do whatever it takes to accomplish a task. Military recruits with different mind-sets and backgrounds work together as one to get the job done. When one set of skills is mastered, a recruit moves forward to conquer another set. Before she knows it, what was once considered impossible is now a reality. This same mind-set can apply to your individual weight-loss goals as well.

Again, the Kingdom of Heaven is like a treasure hidden in the field, which a man found, and hid. In his joy, he goes and sells all that he has, and buys that field.

—Matthew 13:44 (WEB)

FAITH   143

There are two times in life when you will do whatever it takes to get the job done: when you really want something and when you have no choice. Ask for help to embrace the former before you wind up asking for help to survive the latter. You already have all the discipline you could ever need to make this happen. And when you feel like you are running out of discipline, ask God to give you more.

His divine power has granted to us all things that pertain to life and godliness, through the knowledge of him who called us by his own glory and virtue.

—2 Peter 1:3 (WEB)

GOT GUILT?

Feeling guilty about excess weight is a waste of time. This applies to both you and your children. Childhood weight issues can be a very painful topic for parents. Remind yourself that God loves your children more than you, and once you are living a healthy lifestyle, you can help them. Having grown up as an overweight child, I am now privileged to help others lose weight, reminding them that excess weight is a temporary problem. There are tips in chapter 7 on how to help your whole family with weight management, but for now let's focus on the number one way you can help them the most, which is you getting healthy. God is calling you to go forth, not wallow.

You have encircled this mountain long enough.

—Deuteronomy 2:3 (WEB)

BAD GENES?

When looking at pictures of our family members from past generations, most of our ancestors did not have a weight problem. Even if they did, your story is not written yet. Many of my clients are from families with more recent generational weight issues. Most had family members that tried for years to solve the problem with multiple diets, exercise, and even bariatric surgery. If you are going to blame genetics, you need to ask yourself if your family has poor eating habits or maybe considers exercise having to unbuckle a seat belt, get out of the car, and walk in to get a combo meal with a large fry and diet soda. I know what it's like to have fat genes, but by eating the FAITH VS. WEIGHT way, both my clients and I have shut them up, and so can you.

I have worked with international clients who moved to the US from other countries. These were highly educated people who were having a hard time adjusting to an American diet. They were eating like Americans and getting the same results as the rest of us, and sadly, so were their children. On the plus side, when one person gets healthy in the family, it can have a ripple effect. You can set the example and break this curse for your entire family!

GETTING OLD?

We can blame it on aging. However, our kids are the first generation predicted not to outlive their parents unless we get a handle on the obesity epidemic. I will never forget the first time my family and I went to a Six Flags in Texas. It was heartbreaking to see so many obese children in one place. Many of these children were already suffering from obesity-related illnesses. These diseases are not about old age. They are about bad diets. At what age do you lose your spark? The answer is when you give up on your health. At the YMCA, I saw people who were in their sixties and seventies with more energy and zest for life than most forty-year-olds. I remembered one of the ninety-year-olds on a Masters Swim team I used to train with in California posing for a picture with a stack of winning medals around her neck that looked like they weighed more than she did! We now have centenarians competing in marathons! Aging is not the problem. Giving up is the problem.

When it comes to strength, you will lose muscle mass every year past your thirties unless you are doing something to counteract this. You might weigh the same, but you will have more fat than muscle. This is why things "shift." You need some type of resistance training to create the demand for the muscle you are losing. As you age, resistance training is more important than ever. You don't have to bench press three hundred pounds. You just have to work your muscles enough so they are fatigued by the last repetition. Low weights with high reps are a great way to start to avoid joint and ligament injuries/strains in the process. Flexibility also decreases as you age. You do not need a yoga class, but make time to stretch every day. I like to stretch at the end of the day so my muscles are relaxed before sleep.

Power and balance are as simple as throwing a weighted ball for power or practicing standing on one leg for balance. Cardio is obviously a must for your heart. Fast walking counts! If you want to do intervals (going faster every few minutes), make sure you have a steady base of cardio under your belt, meaning you are already able to maintain at least twenty minutes of cardio at an aerobic pace. If you are not there, start where you are and add a few minutes each week.

Just remember you can probably figure out some way to move your body that will benefit your health no matter how old you are, and you may also help a friend in the process. Send out an email and see if any of your buddies are interested. If walking is a struggle, you can use stationary or recumbent bikes. You can also try pool walking. If you like company, check out the Silver Sneakers program with classes across the country for free. You are never too old to take better care of your health to serve the kingdom. People are living longer so keep yourself in good enough shape to enjoy the length of your days. Don't miss out on what might be tomorrow by giving up on today!

The LORD blessed the latter part of Job's life more than the former.

—Job 42:12 (NIV)

Hate Exercise?

I feel your pain. When I was overweight as a child, I was the last person to be picked for any team. I dreaded physical education. At age eleven, I hit puberty (or rather it hit me) because I had reached the magic number of one hundred pounds. It was not pleasant to have to change into gym clothes. No fat kid likes to change into gym clothes. I was also petrified of any sport having anything to do with a ball of any size. I had a negative association with sports and all physical activity. It wasn't until my forties when I started participating and placing in local runs. As I aged, like a tortoise, I started winning because I kept showing up. Many hares hang up their running shoes early. The life lesson here is don't give up. I received my first athletic trophy for a 5K after I turned fifty. It is a plastic trophy that looks like one of the many my children have already amassed. It is the only athletic trophy I have ever received, so it might as well be platinum as far as I am concerned.

> For the vision is yet for the appointed time; It hastens toward the goal and it will not fail. Though it tarries, wait for it; For it will certainly come, it will not delay.
>
> —Habakkuk 2:3 (NASB)

Since many of my clients hate to exercise, we have to figure out a way to make it happen. So we ask God to help us. One of my clients prayed God would not only help her to exercise but that she would actually like it, and now she loves it! First, decide to exercise. Next, choose what type. Then choose your distraction. You might as well use distraction for something worthwhile! Maybe you can't figure out where to start, but perhaps you are an avid book-worm or have certain shows you like. I tell my clients to save their show, or catch up with the news, or read their book during their workout time. If you are a sports fanatic and live games do not coincide with your exercise time, there are thousands of audiobooks on sports that are so motivating you will be sad when your workout is over. Now you will have a positive association with exercise. A stationary bike seems to be the easiest place to start for most, but any aerobic exercise will work. Exercise is a great way to dissipate stress.

Some of you may not need to exercise to lose weight if you really follow the eating plan. But eventually you will have to do some sort of consistent movement if you want a decent shot at a long, healthy life. Not only does exercise help you maintain your goal weight, movement has been linked to longevity. No surprises there. When you exercise, you send your body the message it still needs to keep on trucking. Praise Jesus!

No Time to Exercise?

I have a hard time when people tell me they do not have time to exercise. If heads of state can find time to exercise, so can you. These people don't have time to go to the gym either, but they still make exercise happen. They either exercise at home, work, or in a hotel because it is a priority. They don't exercise because they have time to spare and lack more pressing things screaming for their attention. They are just as busy as the rest of us, if not more so. Assuming people have more time because they have a staff misses the whole point of why they need a staff in the first place.

As for gyms, they are wonderful if you can make it on a regular basis. People who work full-time, commute, and have a family can rarely make it to the gym on a consistent basis unless there is a gym at their work or close to home. In this case, you may need to take your medicine (exercise) in smaller doses. You can split your workouts. You might be able to do a twenty- to thirty-minute quick walk at lunch or up and down the stairwell listening to music on your iPhone. Later you might be able to squeeze in fifteen minutes of resistance training (abdominal crunches, light weights, wall push-ups) in your living room in the evening while you catch up on the news. I have also had my clients pedal on an exercise bike while going through an upper arm routine with short interval bursts (pedaling faster) every three minutes. They finished off with a few abdominal exercises and stretches at the end. Get creative!

When I was stationed in the Washington, DC, Metro area and had the dreaded Beltway commute, I packed my work clothes (uniform) in a gym bag the night before. I also made sure my workout clothes were out and ready to go so I didn't have to wake up any earlier. I drove to work while there was zero traffic and was able to get a workout in during the same amount of time I would have spent commuting. I would then either eat a breakfast (see breakfast/snack chart in the appendix) I had packed the night before, at work or on the way. If I had early-morning meetings, then I worked out at the gym at the end of the day before I went home in order to avoid traffic. Of course I always made sure I had an adequate afternoon snack (see breakfast/ snack chart in the appendix) to power through afternoon workouts and a pre-workout drink (see eating timing and tips) within twenty minutes of the workout, if it had been a while since my snack. A small amount of planning can get you a workout on either end of your workday instead of yet another opportunity to spike cortisol levels and store fat.

Later, as a stay-at-home mom, I had a spin bike in my kitchen. The spin bike landed in my kitchen after I broke my leg skiing. I needed easy access to it when it was time to start using the bike as part of my recovery. It was only supposed to be there on a short-term basis but became a permanent fixture. Everyone wanted to use it! I had to fight for my time on my spin bike! I got over worrying about what this looked like in my kitchen and realized it made perfect sense for my family and me. If I had not had a chance to exercise during the day and was finally getting home after my children's soccer practice, I would sometimes get in an easy workout. At this point, my kids were doing their homework, practicing piano, reading a book, or playing with their media. They did not care if I was sitting on a couch or if I was sitting on a spin bike. If they were engaged in something and not talking to me, then I was listening to an audio book. If they wanted to chat, then we chatted away.

You might be thinking, *I hate bikes*, or *I have no room*, or *I hate to exercise indoors*, or *I'm tired*. Of course I had days I would have rather plopped on the couch or ridden my bike outside on a trail. But my spin bike in the kitchen, which may not have been considered ideal, was one of the main things that helped my recovery, kept me fit, and gave me more energy. This way, I could actually do what I did consider ideal, which was get out on weekend mornings with my family for long, beautiful bike rides. Look at the big picture. A lot of exercise equipment winds up never getting used because it is in a location in the house people are never actually in when they finally have a moment to exercise. If you don't take advantage of the everyday ways to get and stay fit, when the opportunity to enjoy an outdoor fitness outing with your family finally arrives, you may be too out of shape to enjoy it. Instead, make the most of what you've got so you can better enjoy the opportunities you are given.

Even if you have access to a gym, I strongly encourage my clients to have a backup exercise plan at home. Life happens. A stationary bike is a great pick because most people know how to use it and can do it even if they are overweight or have old injuries, within the guidelines of their physician. Bikes are also versatile. At the end of long days when I haven't had a chance to exercise, I like to relax on my bike and pedal with little resistance while I unwind with a book. If it is earlier in the day, then I listen to the Bible and do sprint intervals. If you don't want to invest in exercise equipment, you can download any beginning exercise program app on your cell phone while you are at home. Ask the Holy Spirit for guidance for what will work in your life. It may take a couple of tries. Keep praying for the right idea! Think about this as if your life depended on it because it does. This is a chance for you to focus on how you can make exercise accessible in your life today. Movement is important for longevity. It relieves stress and makes you happy, especially once you start enjoying the endorphins. If you don't have time to exercise, it is time to reprioritize. Preventative health takes less time than disease management.

EATING ON THE RUN

Constant travel, client dinners, and most meals at restaurants do not have to equal weight gain. Believe it or not, you can lose weight when you travel! You may have just conditioned yourself to believe you can't do it. This has nothing to do with the reality of the situation. I am at restaurants more than I like. I always center my meals around a lean protein, vegetables, and a healthy fat. If the restaurant does not have a healthy fat, I have my old standby of hundred-calorie pistachios in my purse. The FAITH VS. WEIGHT diet in the appendix was created for home and travel use.

Participants in executive-level positions are constantly in airports with late-night client dinners, and they too have succeeded with this program. It was designed for people who are on the move. Whether you are in an executive-level position or in the carpool line, you most likely are eating fewer meals at home. This is not ideal, but it does not need to be catastrophic. It is reality, and any program not taking this into account is not going to work in the long run. Even with the challenges of travel, it is not a foregone conclusion you will have excess fat. Travel does not have to equal weight gain. Your mind-set when you travel needs to focus on what will equal weight loss. Just like planning your itinerary, you can do basic planning for your trip to lose weight and improve your health. Besides paying attention to what you eat, figure out at what point in the day you are going to move. The fastest way to get over jet lag is to go for a walk in your new city as early as possible.

FAST FOOD

For breakfast, Starbucks is one of the easiest places to eat somewhat healthy and fast. Try their egg white red pepper bites or a package of single-serve almond butter with a small banana as a midmorning snack. Their protein boxes are a great option as well. Enjoy it with either a green tea or coffee with cinnamon. If it is time for lunch and you want a cheeseburger, then get a single cheeseburger with no sauces and dump the bread. We are not talking a Big Mac. I do the same thing at Chik-fil-A. A grilled chicken sandwich without the bread and a kale salad, removing the sugar-laden cranberries, equals a healthy lunch. At restaurants, grilled items, veggies, and healthy fats are usually easy to find. It is very easy to do this plan on the road. This program has worked from Boston to Berlin.

On vacation, most people are naturally tempted by goodies they don't normally eat at home. They also want to make sure they are getting their money's worth at the buffet. One day of this may be fine for some, but seven days of high-calorie eating on vacation equals the same thing as seven days of high-calorie eating at home. Vacation calories still count. If you are too tempted to walk away from the brunch counters without piling your plate sky high, try ordering from the menu. Oftentimes it is cheaper to order off of the menu instead of paying extra for a large brunch. This may also help you not overdo it. You could also save yourself time and money by having a simple, healthy breakfast such as a hardboiled egg, string cheese, and an apple with almond butter in your room. Instead of expensive brunches and lunches, you can save your funds for eating dinners out at high-quality restaurants. There are always options. Make sure you have your afternoon snack. This way you can at least make a decision with your head instead of your stomach when it comes to dinner. If you wind up at the all-you-can-eat buffet for breakfast, lunch, or dinner, remember just because something is available does not mean you need to overdo it.

TREATS

Save your treat for dessert, which means after dinner, or you will be eating dessert all day. Encouraging clients to have one treat at the end of the day has huge psychological benefits. Even though I recommend keeping your treat to one hundred calories, if you pick a favorite, you will still feel spoiled! When I do have a treat at home, it is usually one black truffle from the company Alter Eco, previously mentioned. Black truffles are made with a small amount of coconut oil, which speeds metabolism, is good for your brain, and reduces hunger. I keep a couple of these in my purse and may have one after dinner at a restaurant or on vacation. You don't always need to order the flaming volcano that feeds ten people. Just because you are at a restaurant or on vacation doesn't mean you need to eat every meal as if it is the Last Supper.

Whenever you can eat at home or prepare your own meals and snacks, take advantage of it. Although snacks on this plan require zero preparation, re-member to grab them before you leave your house or hotel room. When traveling, your afternoon snack can be fruit you pick up at the breakfast buffet at the hotel. I add that to my hundred calories of nuts or nut butters I travel with so I am all set in the afternoon and do not have to go into dinner starving. The right snacks can be your secret weapon at home and on the road. I also travel with my hot cacao mix of one teaspoon of raw cacao and one tablespoon of coconut butter, ready to add to hot water. I enjoy this in the early afternoon. This helps me to not be tempted by all confections all day that will inevitably come my way on any trip.

Incorporate from these suggestions what works for you and dump the rest. Just don't be too fast to dump ideas without trying them before a vacation to see whether or not they help curb cravings at home. If it doesn't work at home, it is not going to work on vacation. Alternatively, if it does work at home, there is no reason it will not work on vacation.

Working Conferences

I always try to have breakfast in my room after I go for a walk in my new city or hit the gym. You can always join others and have a tea or coffee later. When you travel, take advantage of the hotel refrigerator by stocking it with healthy snacks. Most buffet-style breakfasts are loaded with plastic-looking pastries, sugary yogurt, and bagels. You will be happy you ate in your room. With lunches out, you can usually get some protein and a salad with cheese on the side. Avoid starchy carbs and sugary dressings. Ask for olive oil or guacamole. Options are outlined on the FAITH VS. WEIGHT Diet plan for lunch/dinner. For many people who are sugar sensitive, starchy carbs or sugars at breakfast or lunch can cause sugar cravings the rest of the day. Even if you tried to have a virtuous starchy carb at lunch, most likely sugar has been added since restaurant carbohydrates are typically made with sugary sauces, triggering even more cravings. You can avoid these cravings by having your starchy carbs at night.

Unending To-Do Lists

Errands always take longer than expected. The sooner you figure this one out, the more successful you will be. Planning ahead can make or break you. As I write this, my car repairs are taking longer than originally anticipated. Since this is not my first rodeo, I have packed my lunch, just in case. Unfortunately, sitting in the customer waiting area across from me, I noticed a woman polishing off a bag of Fritos. It is 1:30 in the afternoon, and this poor woman already looks worn out. My guess is she did not have lunch and wound up at the vending machine. She is approximately one hundred pounds overweight. I could very easily be in the same position as this woman, from a snack standpoint as well as a weight standpoint. We are no different. The only difference is I have learned the hard way to plan ahead. My choices, her choices, and your choices all add up over time. That's it. If I didn't have my lunch in my small cooler, I still would have had the pistachios in my purse and grabbed the apple sitting out next to the free water bottles. This is not meant to be judgmental. This is meant for you to consider real life options in real-life situations in order to preempt real-life consequences. The choice is yours. Even if you are already in this boat, you can change your destiny starting today.

Running/Extreme Workouts

Many first-time clients tell me they cannot run. This tells me they assume running is a prerequisite to losing weight and keeping it off, but it is not. Although I love to jog, I did not jog for the first time until I was almost eighteen. The majority of my clients do not run. They just keep moving. I share this so you can get it in your head that even though injuries and surgeries may limit your mobility, you can still make the most of what you've got. Although you can always find an appropriate way to exercise, my clients lose weight by changing their diet first. However, I am passionate about people moving because movement is linked to longevity. Just watch what happens when you incorporate both! If you like to run and are not at a manageable weight, then walk, swim, or bike. Why put your joints through the impact of jogging if you have excess weight? This is a great way to get injured. If you want to run, walk first until your weight is manageable. Walk before you run. Nutrition is 80–90 percent of the battle anyway.

Fooling yourself into thinking you are overweight because of the one workout you cannot do will never get you to your goal. Using any intense form of exercise for weight loss is not sustainable. No one will tell you this, but it is true. There will be times in your life when you cannot sustain these effort levels due to injuries, illness, peak times at work, or family situations. If your weight management is dependent on burning nine hundred calories per workout, you will have a problem. If you love to do intense workouts for the sake of doing them and are in the type of shape to handle them, that is a different story. However, I know many people who put on weight when they start running because they think they can justify extra calories, or they wind up getting injured and then stop all forms of exercise. When I was younger, I used to love garlic fries and a banana shake with my mushroom swiss burger after a long run. I realize this may not be everyone else's first pick! However, the point here is my six-mile run may have burned 700–800 calories, while my lunch was well over 1,500, probably pushing 2,000 calories.

When it comes to weight management, many of us still have in our heads the past media sensationalism surrounding overweight people practically killing themselves to lose weight as part of our reality TV. This was demeaning and added to the debasement of human beings in general, but since it makes money, it keeps airing. Even if you do lose weight on an intense program, how long do you think you can continue? Is this your plan for long-term weight management? Sadly, many of these participants are not able to maintain these intense all-day workout programs. If you wind up sidelined, I recommend moving every single day, especially with injuries, illness, peak times at work, and family situations. You don't need to kill yourself, but you do need to move. Do what you can. Fresh air and whatever exercise you can fit in will help you and others through recovery periods. Try to remember to move for at least fifteen minutes after every meal. You will get forty-five minutes of exercise in while helping your body manage blood sugar levels.

I was eighteen when I went through US Navy boot camp. It was hard enough at that age. It is no surprise women in their late thirties and forties attending weekend boot camp classes after sitting at a desk all week are winding up with injuries. No wonder people hate exercise. If you are looking for a training philosophy that will give you the hardest workout for your buck, you need to read a different book. I always ease my clients into their workouts and only challenge them when they are ready, in order to prevent injuries and burnout. Extreme workouts are not a sustainable way to lose weight. As the old saying goes, you cannot out-exercise a bad diet.

Spiked cortisol levels can set the stage for storing fat and creating false hunger. Intense exercise can set you up for this Catch-22. It is not necessary to go to exercise extremes in order to lose weight, and in most cases it is counterproductive. You should always challenge yourself but not stress your body out. Exercise is meant to be invigorating, not an excuse to binge. Months or years of crazy workouts and extreme dieting will deplete your body, leaving you lacking in nutrients that will inevitably lead to cravings. Your body is not craving the cupcake. It is craving real food. Nutritious food and the appropriate amount of exercise are going to eliminate cravings, not create them. Unfortunately, most people just push harder and harder, leaving themselves more depleted and fatter. Extreme diets and workouts will cause you to fail.

I would rather not train a client if they were not open to discussions involving faith, diet, and lifestyle. I have politely fired clients, and clients have politely fired me. You should be on the same page as your trainer. I don't agree with the philosophy of getting your money's worth by not being able to walk the next day; nor should you be inadequately challenged. Still, training is only a small percentage of the equation. Remember, fitness does not start in the gym!

Whether your exercise classes resemble covert military training ops or not doesn't matter. Even if you burn eight hundred calories in a workout, you still need to watch what you eat. How about eating a healthy meal and then going for a bike ride with your family or friends? Another day, you can pick a resistance class like Pilates to build strength. You may burn fewer calories than a Navy SEAL training session, but you will have fewer calories to burn if you are not overdoing it. Too much of our society has the supersize me mentality after boot camp workouts. This is not how the rest of the world maintains their weight, unless they have already adopted our crazy lifestyle. The Mediterranean food pyramid actually has a picture of people dancing. How fun is that? Doesn't look like people torturing themselves to me. When I was stationed in Spain and had the weekend off from work, my friends and I used to dance the night away. I do not remember ever sitting down. There weren't very many chairs. In the evenings, everyone was out and about, from babies in strollers to grandparents. I sadly remember when the first McDonalds came to Jerez, near the town I lived in, off of the Costa De Luz. I often wonder how Americanized their local diet is today.

FASTING AND CLEANSING

I have never seen a person struggling with weight benefit from skipping meals or fasting. As a matter of fact, the female clients at the YMCA who fasted almost always gained weight. Food restriction leads to binge eating.

I realize not everyone who fasts gains weight, and some lose weight. I can only say I have never seen it work as a method for long-term weight management for people who have weight issues. A decrease in energy, muscle mass, endurance, and metabolism seems to be the result. Not much energy left to serve the kingdom! Once I had a client at the YMCA ask me specifically for nutrition help during a long-term fast since this was her religious custom. We devised a weight control plan. She told me this was the first time she did not gain weight during a fast. That being said, there are two benefits of fasting, but the approaches are not the ones most people take. The first applies to weight management, and the second applies to spiritual growth. A best idea for fasting when it comes to weight management with possible brain benefit is fasting for twelve hours between dinner and breakfast.

Your body goes into a ketogenic state to burn fat instead of carbs when you do not eat for several hours. Some research points to potential benefits for your waistline as well as your brain when this occurs. It's easy. All you have to do is stop eating after dinner. This doesn't even feel like fasting. However, you do have to make sure you eat enough during the day, which would mean following the plan. You also have to remember to hydrate during the day. The second benefit is more important than the first and is associated with spiritual fasting. Biblical prayer and fasting is meant for our spiritual growth. It is not intended for vanity purposes; quite the opposite. The whole point of prayer and fasting is to shut out the shouts of outer-world distractions so you can pay attention to God's soft whisper.

> *After the wind there was an earthquake, but the LORD was not in the earthquake. After the earthquake came a fire, but the LORD was not in the fire. And after the fire came a gentle whisper.*
>
> —*1 Kings 19:11–12 (NIV)*

It wasn't until my early thirties that I even considered fasting. I had pretty much decided it wasn't worth the effort until one day a coworker on the basement floor of an old government building lifted the veil from my eyes. I was a young lieutenant, low on the totem pole with all the brass in the Washington, DC, area. My coworker was a lower-grade civil servant, which meant she was not very high on the totem pole either. My first impression of Natalie (not her real name) was not a good one. She didn't strike me as having a strong work ethic. She also didn't seem to be one of the kindest people I had ever worked with. Boy was I wrong. Not only was Natalie a hard worker, beneath her tough-as-nails exterior, she had a heart of gold. Natalie was a grandmother raising her grandbabies because her daughter was checked out on drugs. Contrary to popular belief, not all federal workers are overpaid. She had a meager salary and lived in a high-rise neighborhood known at the time as the murder capital of the US.

One Friday she was more quiet than usual. I found out later she had not eaten that day. Let's just say Natalie was not the dieting kind and would not volunteer this information even if it were the case. When I asked her if she was on a diet, the cleaned-up version of her response was, "Are you nuts? Of course not! It's Good Friday. What kind of a woman would I be if I didn't fast on Good Friday?" And there I was, staring at her like a deer in the headlights. I can tell you exactly what kind of a woman that would be, I thought. That would be me. In my opinion, Natalie's whole life was one big sacrifice. Did she really need to give something else up? She could have had plenty of excuses not to fast, yet, despite her circumstances, she did what she could do to honor the Lord.

For they all put in of their abundance; but she out of her poverty put in all that she had, her whole livelihood.

—Mark 12:44 (NKJV)

Needless to say, since then I've always fasted on Good Friday. If Natalie could do it, so could I. As I grow in my walk with the Lord, I look forward to this day of prayer of fasting, and I always whisper a prayer for Natalie. There really is nothing like prayer and fasting to strip away all of the garbage insulating us from the Lord and from our sisterhood in Christ. Biblical fasting is worth more to those who do it, in the spirit for which it is intended, than any other short-lived positive or negative weight effect. The fasting part is meant to take the focus off of your body, not to be used as a means to abuse it or alter it. Obviously there are many people out there who use fasting as a means for all kinds of things other than what is was biblically intended. Again, I do not recommend you become one of them. If you are spending days fasting for weight loss, you can wind up with more metabolic and psychological damage than when you started. That being said, there is another time we are encouraged to fast.

Referring to a demon possessed boy, Jesus said, "This kind can come out by nothing but prayer and fasting" (Mark 9:29, NKJV).

Sometimes you need the big guns. A day of prayer and fasting can change your perspective overnight as well as help you get rid of some of your own demons.

Since we are on the topic of fasting, we might as well talk about fasting's cousin when it comes to weight loss circles—cleansing. Every morning, I squeeze half a lemon in eight ounces of filtered room temperature water. It is the first thing I drink after brushing my teeth. Lemon in warm or room temperature water has been used for ages as a home remedy cleanse. It also stimulates bile production and gets things moving. Some people who cannot tolerate citrus use green tea or dandelion greens tea. Beyond that, I would not personally purchase a commercially produced cleanse or participate in any cleanse unless it was medically necessary and supervised.

If you really want to cleanse your system, stop eating junk. As you decrease the amount of junk you eat, you give your body a chance to cleanse itself. This is one of the main reasons people feel so much better when they start eating healthy. They are not dealing with the constant sludge of processed foods, and their body is not endlessly struggling with what to do with these foreign invaders. If you drink plenty of water, eat vegetables and fruits, and buy organic, you are cleansing your body. Fiber in fruits, vegetables, and starchy carbohydrates assist your body in performing its own cleansing job. I doubt many centenarians have done a cleanse. If you asked my ninety-five to one hundred-year-old aunts about cleansing, my guess is they would have assumed you were talking about laundry detergent.

Baby Weight to Menopause

What does pregnancy weight have to do with menopause? Many women with grown children tell me they got off track after having kids. Although some are postmenopausal, it is never too late. Fat is just fat: baby fat, menopause fat, divorce fat. It's all just fat. Yes, fat around your abdomen is worse, but again, it is just fat. The same rules of this program apply. This program has helped many postmenopausal women lose fat! Menopause may be a game changer, but it is not a showstopper.

Old Dog? New Tricks!

Maybe childbirth is a distant memory or was not even a part of your journey. You may be retirement planning, not stroller shopping. Either way, you are just too set in your ways to make a change. Why bother? What's the point? It's too hard.

We want instant results. Give yourself time. Just like the invalid, it took us a lifetime to get here. Are we really going to expect to be cured in twenty-four hours? It is normal for you to have a few false starts. Some start the program, and things don't really click until week two or later. By the end of the class, they are the star pupils. At least one woman changed careers to work in the wellness industry because she was so inspired by what she could accomplish through this program. She is one of the people who told me to write this book. The reason this program is seven weeks long is because any new change takes a few weeks to get used to, especially if you need to deal with behaviors that have held you back in the past. Think back to what you have already accomplished in this life. Remember, where you start does not determine where you will finish.

Go to Health!

Losing weight at any age is more about consistent effort than extreme sacrifice. I used to walk with my father when I would visit him at his retirement community. Every time we walked, he would point to at least one person and say, "You see that guy over there? He left fifty pounds on the side of that road, and he's in his eighties." This was my father's way of saying this man or woman started walking after moving to this beautiful golf course community in Florida, and the weight just fell right off. The best part was seeing the T-shirts the residents used to wear that said, "Go to Health!" Having previously lived in South Florida, it was nice to see a suggested expletive that was actually inspiring! You see, my friend, anything is possible! Again, age is not a limiting factor in losing weight or being active. The number of seniors participating in races is on the rise. The number of photographers at many of these events has also increased. One unflattering shot of me at a finish line showed a strained look on my face. The next shot took a broader view with another person in it. Her foot strike across the finish line had the same timing as mine, except she looked completely relaxed. She was in the over-seventy age group. I will look for her at future races. Maybe she can give me some pointers!

Make Your Move

Many women lose faith in exercise while trying to lose weight because they seem to bulk where they don't want to bulk while barely losing any weight. This is because we tend to work the areas we want to lose the hardest. The problem with this approach is that when we work problem areas the hardest, we almost always increase resistance. Increasing resistance builds muscle. It's true you are not going to turn into a heavyweight lifter overnight. However, your muscle will increase in size with heavier resistance. Although this may sound great for your metabolism, we typically eat more than the slight metabolic increase we get. This is why some women are working hard only to find that they are bulking in an area they are trying to minimize while barely losing any weight.

Although you want muscle, women who are losing weight are not looking to increase in size, so how do you work around this? Years ago, high-repetition and low-weight workouts came on the scene. Many saw working out with light weights as a complete waste of time, which is true if you only do the traditional ten to twelve reps. However, if you ensure proper form while increasing the repetitions to twenty or more while increasing speed, you can fatigue the muscle without causing it to significantly increase in size. This is called strength endurance. If you minimize rest in between exercises, your heart rate will be close to a brisk walk, giving your strength routine the added bonus of an easy cardio workout as well. All of my client weight-loss workouts are based on strength endurance. For weight-loss purposes, there is no need to ever lift heavy. Heavy lifting spikes cortisol and increases appetite. This happens when you see women kill it at the gym and then go out for bagels and cream cheese right afterward because they are starving. The same applies to cardio. Cranking up the stair climber to a level 12 is like weightlifting for your legs. Instead, level one or two on an exercise bike pedaling at a faster RPM with three to five-minute intervals of one-minute speed increases is a better way to gain strength endurance without bulking. Here are some exercise tips that will help you work with your body type instead of against it. Consult your physician before starting any exercise plan.

APPLE

(Carry weight in your midsection and upper body.)

Cardio: Your goal is to burn visceral (abdominal) fat. Get on the bike and do interval training. This is the easiest way to burn the most visceral fat. Although Apples can crank up the resistance because they tend not to bulk in their lower body, if you are overweight, I suggest keeping the resistance low and the *RPMs high when doing intervals. If you regularly do cardio, every three to five minutes, just pedal faster for one minute. Do not increase tension. This helps incinerate fat for all body types but is an Apple's best friend! Climb stairs and walk up hills whenever you can! Choose kickboxing over boxing.

Strength: Squats and lunges with no weight are best. Your body weight provides enough resistance. Keep upper body exercises to low weights with high reps since this is where you tend to bulk. Pilates or Bar Method are a great choice. Work on posture. Hula-Hoops are great for your core (try both directions).

PEAR

(Hip width is wider than shoulder width.)

Cardio: Your answer is high rep, low or no resistance for your legs. Fast walking, cycling with zero or low resistance but with high *RPM (this means pedal faster). If you regularly do cardio, every three to five minutes increase speed for one minute, not tension. If you turn up the tension, you may bulk before you start losing, which is exactly what most Pears are trying to avoid. Swimming is a great addition. Avoid stair climbers and hill workouts.

Instead, walk faster with no incline. No need to jog unless you enjoy it. Choose boxing instead of kickboxing. Keep resistance low in spin class.

Strength: I still recommend low weights with high reps. However, you can incorporate body moves for your upper body. Push-ups (modified included) are a great addition. Modified pull-ups and chin-ups are also a great addition. Limit lunges, squats, and mountain climbers. Best leg exercises are sets of leg lifts (forward, side, and back). High reps with twenty minimum per set.

Hourglass

(Chest and hips are similar width, and waist is smaller.)

Cardio: Your answer is high rep, low or no resistance for your entire body. Fast walking, jogging (not sprinting), cycling with zero or low tension but with high *RPM (that means pedal faster). If you add resistance, you may bulk before you start losing, and typically you are trying to avoid this. Avoid stair climbers and hill workouts. Swimming is great! Choose boxing over kickboxing.

Strength: Keep upper and lower body resistance to low weights with high reps. Minimize lunges, squats, and mountain climbers. Best leg exercises are sets of leg lifts (forward, side, and back). High reps with twenty minimum per set.

*RPM = revolutions per minute

Rectangle

(Chest, hips, and waist are similar in measurements.)

Cardio: Same as hourglass until you reach your goal weight. Once you reach your goal, pick whatever exercise you enjoy and go for it. Your weight/muscle increases tend to evenly distribute.

Strength: Start with low weights with high reps for your total body until you reach goal. Once you reach your goal, you can increase load as you are comfortable with your weights and your results. Make sure you do oblique moves to create a waist. Think about adding a Pilates class. Hula-Hoops are great for your core (try both directions). Keep in mind, strenuous exertion does increase cortisol, which increases a host of other things, including weight. No need to overdo it.

BALANCE, POWER, AND FLEXIBILITY

Balance: Practice getting on and off a Bosu at the gym. At home or at the gym, stand on one leg, doing various leg lifts with the other. This also improves core strength.

Power: This is explosive strength. Think throwing a weighted ball, which is a fun way to mix things up. Boxing and kickboxing are power workouts.

Flexibility: Yoga is great, but if you barely have time to do cardio and strength, at least completely stretch before bed.

FOR EVERY BODY

Invest in an exercise bike for home use and a few light weights. This is a no-brainer. I cannot tell you how many people never make progress because they are unable to make it to the gym for a week or for a month! Learn to adapt to unpredictable schedules, making exercise a priority is key!

Pilates and Bar Method are a great choice for everyone, but they can especially make a difference for Apples and Rectangles.

Pay attention to your heart rate to make sure that you are not overdoing it.

Never look at exercise alone as a way to lose weight. As we age, we are not able to do enough in order to influence the scale. However, when combined with the right kind of eating, exercise does help people maintain weight loss. It also has impact beyond the physiological ones of controlling blood sugar, improving brain health, strengthening bones, and helping your heart. Exercise increases your vitality! It is a fountain of youth providing you with mobility and agility. It can also provide a confidence boost when losing weight if you choose the right exercises described for your particular body type.

Take a Stand

I will never forget one group in particular I facilitated at the YMCA. A participant was going through a nasty divorce and came to class every week looking like she was at the end of her rope. I wondered how she even mustered enough energy to get in her car at the end of her long workday, drive in traffic, and then climb the stairs to class. She never smiled. In the meantime, most of the class was making steady progress and reporting their victories. Although this woman did not seem to be overtly making progress, she kept showing up. One day, she opened up about another woman in the cubicle next to her who had a candy jar on her desk and always "pushed" her to eat it so she would "feel better." At least this woman was now participating, but she still did not seem to be reaping any real benefit from the class. Over time, most of the class was understanding but did not expect great changes from this woman. Then one day she came in with a huge smile and a take-charge attitude toward life. She looked so different. I realized that was because I had never seen her smile! She announced she had slowly started following the healthy eating plan and was losing weight. Obviously she had not lost a significant amount of weight, since she had just started, but her entire demeanor had changed. She told her coworker, "Thanks but no thanks," and announced she was done overdoing sugar. She was sick and tired of being sick and tired. Everyone in the class was speechless. She appeared to be the least likely to succeed, yet her progress continued. Then another classmate perked right up and said, "If she can do it, I can do it too!" And she did. Now we were all smiling.

Love Your Neighbor

You need faith in order to believe you can make permanent lifestyle changes toward a healthier you. Ask the Lord to increase your faith in your ability to positively influence your own health and eventually those around you. Not having faith affects your neighbor. We have all been through times where we needed someone else to have faith in us when we didn't. Sometimes we need to see people having faith in the Lord Jesus Christ in their own area of struggle. The lady described above kept coming back even before she thought she was going to make any changes. She saw others asking the Lord for help in order to make progress. She started having faith in the process, but first she had to see others benefitting from their faith for her to make progress. She had to hear them tell their stories. Eventually, she influenced the rest of the class. Faith can be contagious. If you and I don't have enough faith as Christians to take care of our bodies, who will?

CHANGE YOUR LIFE

WEEK THREE: FAITH

*So we fix our eyes not on what is seen, but on what is unseen, since
what is seen is temporary, but what is unseen is eternal.*

—2 Corinthians 4:18 (NIV)

FOR YOUR SOUL

Do the choices you make reflect your faith in your ability to lose weight? If
not, examine whether or not you have faith in this area. If you are struggling,
ask for a double portion of faith!

Do you have the kind of faith that would touch Jesus in a crowd? If not, take
steps to increase your faith. Start with listening to the Bible. It is the greatest
story ever told about faith.

When you examine your doubts, can you see how these may be lies planted
by the enemy?

When you examine your faith, can you see times in the past where your faith
manifested itself in truth?

Can you see how your level of faith is directly impacting your decisions today
as well as tomorrow?

Do you believe what the Bible says about faith? Do you still believe it when
it comes to your weight?

Are your foregone conclusions holding you back?

Faith is contagious, *and so is doubt*. Notice how your faith affects others.

For Your Body

For weight loss: Healthy eating is number one. Movement is second but extremely necessary for good health and weight management.

For longevity, do resistance training and mix in some interval cardio.

If you are not exercising already, write down three possibilities. Now write down three ways you might better enjoy your time while doing them. Ask God to help you like exercise.

Exercise for your body type to start seeing results.

Do you have a backup exercise plan at home in an area of the house that is accessible when you need it?

You gain weight on the road the same way you do at home. No longer allow travel to be an excuse. This doesn't mean you cannot ever have a small sample of a treat or specialty of the house as a dessert. You just can't do it for seven days, three meals a day, and wonder why you are not making progress. Have a little at the end of each day for dessert as part of your plan. Save it for the last day of vacation or travel if this tends to be an issue.

Justice

Yet the Lord longs to be gracious to you; therefore he will rise up to show you compassion. For the LORD is a God of justice. Blessed are all who wait for him!

—*Isaiah 30:18 (NIV)*

Whether you are a Christian or not, you may feel, as do others, that justice is not served on many levels. This unresolved tension triggers anxiety leading to unhealthy compulsive behaviors, including overeating. Ultimately, this is a question of trust. Do you trust God or not? This verse tells us "the Lord is a God of justice." We can trust him. There is no room for interpretation. Yet the man-made suffering we see in this world on a daily basis seems to reveal a different story. So which is it? Can we trust God will bring justice out of these wrongs or not? If we look at justice with only our human understanding, we have clearly lost the battle. From a human perspective, we are viewing justice as if looking at a single photograph. It is as if we are frozen in time, instead of seeing time as a continuum. If we look at justice from an eternal perspective, we see the entire movie, from beginning to end. Justice was served on the cross simultaneously affecting our past, present, and future. Whether we see it or not, justice was, is, and will always be served. It may not be served in the way we expect it, or even in our lifetime, but it will be served.

Your job is to put your need for God above your need for justice. Satan's job is to put your need for justice above your need for God, making it easier for you to justify an unhealthy behavior. He wants you to believe God is the one treating you or others unjustly, just like he did with Eve. If you do not trust God's justice, you will not trust God. A lack of trust makes you anxious, ultimately inhibiting your ability to make healthy choices. The more you trust God, the more you are at peace, making it easier to relax, positively affecting your health.

> *And those whom He predestined, He also called; and those whom He called, He also justified; and those whom He justified, He also glorified.*
>
> *—Romans 8:30 (MEV)*

Justice belongs to God. He may or may not handle justice in a way you understand, but it is still His department. Many people's lives are so focused on waiting for their version of justice to be served for something that happened in the past they wind up not treating themselves or others justly today. Since justice has already been taken care of, it is a waste of time to focus on someone else's sin, since we can do nothing about their sin except the one thing we are called to do, which is to forgive. As for your own house, you can focus on God's glory and let God focus on justice. Focusing on His glory instead of your need for justice inspires you to live a healthier life. Ironically, we are all called to be a part of His plan for justice, helping others to deal with injustices, as part of loving our neighbor, not for our need for justice. If we are hyper focused on our need for justice, we will miss His glory. In the meantime, you have your own set of instructions:

> *He has shown you, O mortal, what is good. And what does the LORD require of you? To act justly and to love mercy and to walk humbly with your God.*
>
> *—Micah 6:8 (NIV)*

"Act justly" applies to others as well as to yourself. There is no fine print saying, "Do this only if you feel all of your injustices have been resolved to your satisfaction." If you continually compare your life to everyone else's and feel God is being unjust, you will not act justly to others or to yourself. Resentment will surface. Even small resentments can add up over time, seriously affecting your health and your relationships. Resentment can also keep you fat and even harden your heart. Instead of believing everyone else has it better, let's trust God to do His job while we do ours. Stop blaming others' current or past injustices for your unhealthy behaviors. Focus on what the Lord requires of you instead. There will be less waiting, and wasting of time, for all parties involved.

Love the Lord Your God

Trusting God positively affects your health. Studies show fewer anxiety-related health conditions in those who participate in faith-based activities. If you are still struggling with letting current or past injustices go, ask yourself if you are struggling with trusting God. My guess is yes. Whether or not you are at peace when it comes to God's ideas on justice will depend on whether or not you are at peace with God. As you grow in your faith, you will find greater peace. Some people seem to have a gradual progression with their faith while others are all-in from the start—just as there are people who read the Bible as if it were just another history book, or work of fiction, while others read it and put their complete trust in Jesus overnight. It is the same book, so why the different outcomes?

SOWING THE SEEDS OF LOVE

In the parable of the sower, Matthew, chapter 13, Jesus talks about four different types of people and their *state of heart* upon hearing God's Word. In this case, God's Word is a seed. Depending on the condition of one's heart, God's Word will either "bloom where it is planted" or not. For simplicity sake, I have categorized each heart condition related to one's faith. In some cases, there may be zero correlation between someone's faith or lack of it when it comes to their weight. However, it is just as easy to see how someone's faith could affect everything from their perception of justice to weight management and beyond.

A HEART CONDITION

Hardened heart: someone who is dead to sin. Matthew, chapter 13, talks about birds, which are in this case Satan, eating up all of the seeds before any of them can take root. This person tries to take justice into their own hands because they don't trust anyone else to do it, especially not God. Obviously there is no real faith or trust in God. (For the record, many hardened hearts have later gone on to bear much fruit, so keep praying if you are struggling with or are dealing with someone in this category.) From a health perspective, you may find this person has already given up or may even be fanatical in their commitment to either a very strict diet or gluttony.

Shallow heart: the people who fall under this category are very excited about their newfound faith when they first hear the Word of God, but as soon as they have to take a stand, they run for the hills. This seed falls on rocky ground with an initial growth spurt and then dies because of a lack of nourishment. This person tends to blame everyone else for injustices, even the ones they could have positively influenced for the better. This person may start out with a bang when it comes to committing to the latest diet but quickly fizzles out.

Distracted heart: this is someone who is too busy to commit regularly to spending time with God developing her faith. We are all busy, right? What we don't realize is we are the only ones who can prioritize our to-do lists. No one else can do this for us. Because there is always something more pressing, this seed's growth gets choked out by other priorities, potentially leading to a hardened heart. This person is running away from past and current injustices instead of leaving them at the foot of the cross. They may tend to focus on the next latest diet craze while still on their current diet, most likely distracted by someone else's progress.

Whole heart: This seed is not just surviving, it is thriving, and it bears much fruit. The possibility for its growth is multiplied "a hundred, sixty, or thirty times." I find the order of this numbering interesting. We usually start from lowest to highest. This passage starts with the highest expectation first. Miracles can happen through this heart of faith, because it is unequivocally born again. This is where you will see God's glory. This person is not focused on their need for justice. This person is focused on helping others who suffer injustices while also cultivating seeds of faith. However, this person can be guilty of putting the needs of others over their own health, ultimately running out of gas. Although they are aware their body is to be used for God's glory, they may not know the best way to take care of it or make it a big enough priority. They have to be reminded that in order to love their neighbor as themselves, they have to love themselves.

I will give you a new heart and put a new spirit in you; I will remove from you your heart of stone and give you a heart of flesh.

—*Ezekiel 36:26 (NIV)*

What is your diagnosis? If you are not yet where you would like to be when it comes to your faith, ask the Lord to remove your "heart of stone and give you a heart of flesh." A heart of flesh loves like Jesus. It also needs to be loved in return, since it has a great compassion for suffering. Remember to pray for others who need a heart of flesh, especially the person you want to see brought to justice. If they already had faith, they probably wouldn't have wound up on your Most Wanted poster for justice in the first place.

Change Your Brain

The symbol for justice is a balanced scale. Treating others how you want to be treated is the underlying message. This section explores these three areas of justice regarding your health:

Thou shalt not covet thy neighbor's skinny jeans.

Forgive as the Lord has forgiven you, whether you believe justice was served or not.

Love yourself as much as you love your neighbor so you can love more neighbors.

1) Thou shalt not covet thy neighbor's skinny jeans.

If your biggest health complaint is you cannot eat whatever you want and fit into a pair of skinny jeans, it's time to get on your knees and thank God. There are people unable to get out of hospital beds who would gladly trade places with you. Often, I have to remind new clients who are discouraged with their bodies that they were able to walk into the classroom or fitness facility, and God willing, they will walk out. What a blessing. Do you appreciate what your body can do, or do you despise it? Your body is a gift from God. How would you feel if you gave someone a gift lovingly handmade especially for him, and he hated it or trashed it? Remember to thank God for His handmade gift. What other tangible remnant do you have that God specifically made for you other than your body that He blew the breath of life into? If you have given birth or attended one, you know the excitement of a first breath. Your body with God's breath allows you to do whatever He is calling you to do today. This is why you have a body. Work on what you can do to love the gift of your body rather than obsessing over nonsense you cannot control. Many have genetic issues causing far worse problems than packing on a few pounds after polishing off one too many doughnuts. Of the problems to have, this is workable. This is actually a wonderful problem to have since it at least gets us thinking about our health before it's too late. Everyone has some problem area they need to work on. He is certainly bigger than your biggest problem.

"God, if I can't be skinny, please give me fat friends." I used to see this sign in Christian bookstores. It made me want to laugh and cry at the same time. Before FAITH VS. WEIGHT, I led and participated in a few Bible study groups in different parts of the country. Many times we prayed for someone's diabetes or one of the other chronic lifestyle, obesity-related health issues for a member in our group. Then we immediately plowed into the weekly potluck table filled with lemon bars, brownies, cookies, and chips. It's like the cause and effect of eating unhealthy foods in large quantities was as far away from contributing to these health problems as the east is from the west. Still I could almost hear the words of Jesus in my head saying, "Do you want to be healed?" Alrighty, so I guess I won't be invited to your next potluck! Unfortunately, overdoing it with food goes on nonstop at social gatherings all over the country and often leads to overdoing it with exercise for those who are so inclined. What we really crave is fellowship. Unhealthy decisions do not need to be a part of fellowship. You may watch others and think, *Hmm, she can eat chocolate cake and fried chicken and still be a size 2*, but what you may not see is the rest of her daily total calorie consumption and activity level. Or maybe she just has the type of genes where a higher percentage of her calories go to muscle instead of fat.

I remember many mornings when I was sixteen years old sitting across from my pencil-thin brother who would down four doughnuts for breakfast as I was trying to lose weight. I would slurp on a straw stuck in the latest diet shake, hoping to suck down the last drop because I was starving. I was unaware that these diet shakes spiked my blood sugar, leaving me hungrier than before I started, while also leading to all-day sugar cravings! Although we had healthy dinners, the rest of the day was a free-for-all. Many high school girls are going through far worse heartbreak and drama when it comes to their diets today. The lesson learned here is you must start with real food and continue to eat it throughout the day. One meal a day of real food is not enough to offset a day of eating junk even if what you are eating and drinking is labeled "diet."

Healthy eating starts with breakfast. Blood sugar control, or lack of it, begins in the morning. The earlier this is ingrained in families, the less chance there is of weight issues later. Adding real food containing protein and cutting back on sugar and excess carbohydrates, especially refined carbohydrates, is a great place to start with all meals, especially breakfast. It doesn't matter what everyone else is eating. You have to do what works for you. Some people have more muscle or more of certain type of hormones, a faster metabolism, or a body that processes carbohydrates and fats differently, or they are an ultra-marathon runner. Stop worrying about everyone else "and walk humbly with your God" (Micah 6:8 NIV).

Skinny does not necessarily equal healthy. Some people who are underweight are so caught up in their work or stressed out they forget to eat, and they are thin, while others living the same scenario are fat. Many also assume skipping meals might help with weight loss because their thin friend skips breakfast. Skipping meals or fasting usually backfires as a method for weight control for those who have weight issues. In some cases, it can negatively affect a diabetic's blood sugar.

I am not a clinician or a researcher, but I do know there are plenty of books on everything you could ever want to know about metabolism. Yet we have barely scraped the surface. Even with all this knowledge, we are still fat. This is because we are looking for an answer telling us something different from what we already know: what you eat and drink matters. Even if you are a size 0 and could eat whatever you wanted or if researchers came up with a pill allowing you to eat chocolate-covered doughnuts all day and you did not gain an ounce, you still need energy from real food. You are called to take care of your body. If not, your body will not take care of you. Food is wasted when you throw it away, but it's a greater waste when you eat more than you need, especially when it comes to junk. Heart disease, diabetes, metabolic syndrome, and gout are debilitating and expensive. Realize sooner, before you have no choice later, that all roads lead to a healthy, real food diet.

Use the Common Sense God Gave You

You and I are not so-and-so. We cannot eat fried chicken and doughnuts whenever we feel like it and not gain weight. If you and I were so-and-so, then you would not be reading, and I would not be writing this book. Maybe you used to be so-and-so and hit menopause, or sitting at a desk all day is finally catching up. Either way, it is genetically predetermined where fat will be deposited on your body, and certain foods cause the body to store fat more easily. In most cases, this equals pounds where you are already the most self-conscious. Skip food that is not calorie worthy and use your calories to provide maximum energy. Wasting calories is like wasting money because both lead to regret.

Nature versus Nurture

Nature (genetics) is what you received at birth, while nurture is what you do with it. Since you are still walking around on this planet, thank God for having good genes! However, it is still up to you to take care of them. Even if you had happened upon skinny genes, you would find there is still a wide birth as to where you could wind up in terms of your weight and overall health. I had a childhood friend who was definitely the slim one of the two of us. As adults, I had always weighed twenty to fifty pounds more than she did, depending on what age and stage of life I was in. She always looked as if she had stepped off the runway and had participated in several beauty pageants. She was literally a beauty queen. Even pregnant, she gained the minimal amount of weight, whereas I was at the maximum end recommended for my height with both of my pregnancies. However, when we reconnected recently, she gave me a pair of jeans that no longer fit her. All I could think was that there was no way her jeans were going to fit me. At least that is how it was when we were teenagers. Then I tried on the jeans, and to my shock, they were too big. She said, "I will never be that weight again," as if it were a done deal. By the intensity of her tone, I could tell this discussion was closed and that she had already given up. I could sense the resignation in her voice, and my heart grieved for her. This had nothing to do with weight. This had to do with her lack of faith in her ability to lose the weight. Although for most of my life weight had been a struggle, I never realized there was an option to throw in the towel. Have you already given up? If you have already decided you will never lose your excess pounds, you will prove yourself right. Unfortunately, my friend has gained more weight since that visit.

If you don't get a handle on your current weight, most likely you will gain more. This is because your body composition will shift from less muscle to more fat because of inactivity, diet, or aging, unless you do something to reverse this trend. Take the offense instead of defense in your overall health and weight battle. Whether you were born with skinny genes or not, sooner or later most women and men have to exert extra energy to win this war. From a health perspective, even good genes can only go so far. Whether you believe you have fat genes or not, you want to encourage positive genetic interactions while discouraging negative ones with your lifestyle, not in spite of it.

2) Forgive as the Lord has forgiven you ... whether you believe justice was served or not.

"For my thoughts are not your thoughts, neither are your ways my ways," declares the LORD.

—Isaiah 55:8 (NIV)

What happens when you feel justice is lacking? Do you numb yourself with food because you don't see a resolution to a local or global injustice? Maybe it is more personal. Someone got away with something, and you or someone you love is left with a lifetime of pain. In the windmills of your mind, you may still be playing out injustices over and over again, making them seem immortal. The truth is nobody gets away with anything. Still, the feelings of desperation, sadness or loss accompanied by prolonged agonies may tempt you to ask, why bother? In many cases, there are no earthly resolutions to heavenly battles. You will only find peace if you stop wasting your time looking for one. Ask for healing while trusting God to make a way where there is none. Even in the cases where justice is served according to human laws, the pain doesn't automatically go away! It won't go away until you learn how to forgive. Here is where allowing the Lord's graciousness and compassion to begin their job of healing comes in. Jesus did not come to teach justice. He came to teach forgiveness. You need to forgive as much as you need forgiveness. Since Jesus states you are going to be forgiven in the same way you forgive, you have great incentive to practice forgiveness.

ABUSIVE RELATIONSHIPS

There is an inordinate number of injustices, but abusive relationships seem to be one of the most prevalent. If you are in an abusive relationship, you are not alone. You are also only one phone call away from help. The National Domestic Abuse hotline is 1-800-799-SAFE. There are also many agencies available that will confidentially provide food, clothing, and a place to stay as well as free legal advice. You can literally walk out the door right now with your kids and the clothes on your back. There is hope, but you have to take the first step.

The LORD will fight for you; you need only to be still.

—Exodus 14:14 (NIV)

My brother and I were born into an abusive household. What started out as verbal abuse from my father later became physical when my mother was pregnant with her first child, which happened to be me. Eleven years later, my mother was able to end this cycle of abuse by leaving with her children. Her faith in God was the only thing that allowed her to do this. It was all she had left. Like most abused women, she had very low self-confidence. The goal of the abuser is to break their victims down physically, emotionally, and psychologically. Why do women stay in these relationships? By manipulation and fear, also known as "false evidence appearing real," the abuser convinces his victim there is no way out. Since low self-esteem is already present, the victim doubts she deserves any better. This psychological state is almost more disturbing than the fear.

Confronting these situations are often life-or-death scenarios for all involved, even the abuser. In our case, which is not atypical, it saved my mother's life and taught me that my life did not have to take the same turn. My mother went on to accomplish many great things. My brother, who is a blessing to society, has a joyful home life with his wonderful wife and six kids. The bottom line is that a generational curse was broken. It eventually saved my father's life as well, although he did not see it that way at the time.

It is easy to portray an abuser like my father in the worst possible light. This is where the paradox of forgiveness comes in. My father was raised in Italy during the era of Mussolini and World War II. His father lost his vision working in coal mines, requiring my father to leave school after fifth grade in order to tend to the family farm. Needless to say, these were harsh times. As a young child, my father remembered helplessly watching his grandfather stabbing his mother over a land dispute. Because his father was limited in his capacity to protect both my father and grandmother, my father lived in a constant state of fear. As a young boy, he was repeatedly physically abused by one of his four older brothers. Later on in life, he would have nightmares, remembering these instances or the air raids he experienced as a child. My father did not talk much about his childhood because he had no desire to relive it. Italy was not a destination location for him. Although my father's childhood in no way justified him abusing my mother, the point here is hurt people hurt people. Eventually, a stronghold of generational violence was shattered in him as well. By accepting grace through the precious blood of the Lord Jesus Christ, my father was set free. Sadly, this did not happen until years after my mother left him, but at least it happened.

If you are using injustice as a reason to seek comfort through overeating, ask God for help. How do you get past all of these hurts in order to move on? You must forgive your neighbor. I realize this is easier said than done. I have asked the Lord to supernaturally help me to forgive when I could not, and He has done this for me on more than one occasion. You may be afraid to forgive because forgiveness makes you feel vulnerable. Yet you cannot have new life without it. What we don't understand is we are vulnerable whether we choose to forgive or not. We are either vulnerable to God when we forgive or vulnerable to the person who hurt us. Only one leads to fullness of life.

3. Love yourself as much as you love your neighbor … so you can love more neighbors.

> *He will make your righteousness go out as the light, and your justice as the noon day sun.*
>
> *—Psalm 37:6 (WEB)*

If you don't bask in the illuminating light of Christ's love, you will look for love elsewhere. This is why it is so important for women of all ages to have their identity in Christ. By not loving and accepting God's love first, you can wind up seeking acceptance from the wrong people, or in some cases from the right people but in the wrong ways. Because of this, many women become people pleasers. Although you are supposed to love your neighbor, becoming a people pleaser is not what God intended.

> *As Jesus and his disciples were on their way, he came to a village where a woman named Martha opened her home to him. She had a sister called Mary, who sat at the Lord's feet listening to what he said. But Martha was distracted by all the preparations that had to be made. She came to him and asked, "Lord, don't you care that my sister has left me to do the work by myself? Tell her to help me!" "Martha, Martha," the Lord answered, "you are worried and upset about many things, but few things are needed*
>
> *—or indeed only one. Mary has chosen what is better, and it will not be taken away from her."*
> *—Luke 10:38–42 (NIV)*

Martha was running around with the daily grind and didn't have time to simply sit down and absorb Jesus's teachings. Jesus gently reminded her that this was precisely why she was worried about so many things! This describes how most of us live today.

She was ignoring her spiritual needs by doing all of the right things while also making sure she was getting the credit. You can't shine the light of Christ if you don't spend time at the foot of the cross or if you are worried about who is getting the credit. This is true even if you are doing all of the "right" things!

It is a constant battle with pride not to chase humankind's approval. It takes discipline to live internally with a focus on the Lord rather than everyone else's applause. However, you will never find your calling if you continue to chase humankind's approval. You will also not be at peace until you use your gifts the way God intended. Once you are fully engaged in doing what you were created to do, it really doesn't matter who gets the credit.

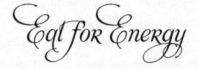

Common sense is not so common.

—*Voltaire*

We often hear people talk about fat genes and what an injustice it is if they happen to be the recipient of them. I can clearly see in my own family who did and did not inherit them. However, if you look at old photographs of your family in the early 1900s, you might see a different picture. When I see old photographs of my family on both sides, there were no weight issues. I am guessing this is because they were farmers and had to physically work for their food. It wasn't until the introduction of processed foods that we saw weight issues emerge. This should tell us something. We saw how some gained weight eating the same processed foods as others, yet they were not affected in the same way.

The first time I realized the effects of different food choices (with approximately the same number of calories) was after my parents' divorce when I was eleven. Initially, I went to live with my mother, who was struggling to work as a teacher in the day and completing her master's degree at night. We lived off of the local burger drive-through. By high school, my brother and I went to live with our father, who was disabled due to a work accident. Fortunately, he enjoyed cooking, and he cooked every day. His love for the Italian food of his childhood was one of the few happy memories he had growing up, and because of this, he prepared mostly Mediterranean meals for us. During the summer, we ate almost all of our meals at home. No longer subsisting on fast food, the excess weight came off. This was round one.

At various times in my life, I went back and forth with weight gain. Whenever I started eating the standard American diet (SAD), I packed on the pounds. I was not immune to the free-for-all of fast-food living in college and gaining the freshman fifteen. The same thing happened when I gained another fifteen pounds returning to the states after being stationed in Spain. My answer to losing weight in those days was to just workout harder.

However, later in life, pregnancy brought on different challenges. With each child, I gained fifty pounds. At the time, my husband traveled for work, and I had limited time to exercise. Since I couldn't burn the calories working out, I was left with only one option, which was to eat healthier. At forty years old with a newborn and two-and-a-half-year-old, I wondered if I would ever get back to my pre-pregnancy weight. It turned out that being limited in time to exercise helped me to realize that nutrition trumped exercise when it came to losing weight, especially in the short term. This was a new concept for me. It didn't mean that exercise did not matter. It just meant that what I put in my mouth mattered more than I had realized. With real food and moderate exercise, you will also find your happy medium. Treating your body justly means balancing food and exercise.

This lesson came home once again when I broke my leg skiing in Canada. Back in our hotel room on the second day of our vacation, barely able to see out of the snow blanketed window, I realized I was facing about a year before I would be running any kind of distance again. I was alone in the room, or so I thought. It turned out I had company. Staring me right in the face were the Rocky Mountain Chocolate Factory Christmas chocolates we had bought for our kids for Christmas. Let me tell you how easy it would have been to face-plant into the kid's Christmas chocolates! Then as clear as day, the Holy Spirit reminded me that although I had one problem with my broken leg, if I dove into those chocolates, I would now have two. This, my friend, is the crux of this book. This was the first time I remember making a conscious decision not to use food for comfort. I wouldn't have given it a second thought up until that point. I proceeded to yell at the Rocky Mountain Chocolate Factory Christmas chocolates, telling them I was not going down without a fight, to which they appeared disinterested. Of course, I blame my outburst on the painkillers. The point is it had finally dawned on me: if I had one chocolate pity party, it would have led to another and then another with no end in sight.

It's Just Not Fair

If you are suffering with an injury or disease, it is even more important to eat healthier. You need the right fuel for energy and recovery. The problem is that this is precisely the time we want to sulk in our sea salt caramel. Many view the fact that they are injured or have a disease as unfair. This is human nature. However, I promise you that this mind-set will guarantee failure. Instead of sulking, I teach my clients not to think of missing out but instead to pick their favorites. This applies to their time as well as their food choices. I was able to catch up on reading. As for food, if you pick your favorite as a small dessert, this makes saying no to 90 percent of the other processed junk and subsequent pity parties a lot easier. The candy at the checkout and the stale birthday cake may not even be close to being a favorite, so why bother. Over time, the favorites I choose now tend to create energy instead of robbing it, because energy is one of my favorite things! I suggest you identify at least one favorite you can have in small amounts and have it as your dessert, ideally keeping it to one hundred calories, especially if you are going through a time of recovery. Tell yourself you can have one hundred calories' worth every day for as long as you want, and see if this helps. Although many do not have a specific caloric limit, a small dessert is the approach most Europeans take. It is not in excess that you are satisfied but in knowing you can have it if you want it as long as you can be temperate with it. Identifying a few favorite foods helps you set boundaries.

Highs and Lows

After sixteen years of active and reserve duty with the navy, I was ready to try something "girly," so I became a fashion consultant in the San Francisco Bay Area. Of the two hundred beautiful customers I served, I remember only about seven of them being happy with their bodies. I wanted women to feel better about themselves from the inside out, not the other way around. While I was a fashion consultant, I learned what the phrase "high/low" meant when it came to fashion. An example might be to pair a higher-cost designer outfit with a lower-cost tank top from a discount retailer. I am a huge fan of the fashion high/low principle not just because of the bang for the buck but also for the limitless possibilities for creativity. It is never boring. You can still find me at consignment shops or at a mall booth buying $5.99 jeggings to go with a designer vest. As a fashion consultant, most of my outfits were on the high end with the occasional low-end accent. Too much low, and I could have wound up looking shabby, which was not good for business.

I recommend the same approach when it comes to eating. Every day, the majority of your meals should be on the high end nutritionally. By high, I do not mean expensive; I mean real quality food. Real food is delicious and satisfying. Contrary to popular belief, it does not take more time. It often takes less. However, if you do wind up at the drive-through, you can still get a grilled chicken salad. You can add a favorite on the low end if the majority of your meals are on the high. Think of a low-end food item as you would an accent item in fashion, similar to a scarf paired with an outfit. Remember to limit the amount of low-end foods or you will wind up looking shabby as well!

As for prepared meals, shakes, and bars, I would love to tell you that you could buy a prepared meal (frozen dinner), shake, or bar with the same protein, fat, fiber, and carbohydrate combination recommended on the FAITH VS. WEIGHT plan and be done with it. However, even if processed foods did not cause the roller-coaster ride of cravings previously discussed, they have other drawbacks. Either they do not take up the same volume in your stomach, leaving you hungry, or your body cannot break down the foreign ingredients easily since it doesn't recognize them, leaving you with less energy. Worst-case scenario, if you are in a situation where your meal planning is a train wreck, you can use this tip I learned many years ago when I served in the navy drug and alcohol rehabilitation program. Overeaters Anonymous was another one of the addiction programs offered. The head of this Navy program at the time would put his hands together similar to the Allstate logo and say, "This is your stomach. You don't need more food than this at any one time." This was a powerful, yet simple reminder not to overdo it, especially when the choices are less than ideal.

I Know Exactly What I Am Missing

Justice is sticking up for yourself even when the threat appears to be benign. Often, someone who doesn't know me will kindly offer me a sugary treat and act shocked when I politely turn it down. This is because our culture supports eating sugar nonstop all day. The next words out of their mouth are, "You have no idea what you are missing!" Then they offer it again out of a sense of hospitality. I graciously decline, again. This usually happens in a social or office setting. However, the places notorious for passing out food products are coffee shops and grocery stores. Do yourself a favor and skip the samples unless you want to be derailed for the rest of the day. Anytime you have sugar, you are potentially waking up your personal sugar monster! When I decline doughnuts at 10:00 a.m. or cookies at 3:00 p.m., the only thing I am missing out on is an extra few hundred calories and craving more sugar for the rest of the day. I am also missing out on feeling sluggish. I do not need to eat of every tree in the garden, and neither do you. So, yes, I know exactly what I am missing!

Eating at nonscheduled meal and snack times has very little to do with actually wanting food. If it did, then you would have a salad instead of a cookie. It has more to do with avoiding the feeling that you are missing out on something, which can be perceived by some as an injustice. If everyone else is having one, why can't you? If you operate under that thinking, you will also wind up with everyone else's health ailments. There will be no lack of food products to try in your future. Every day, food manufactures are coming up with the next best thing to get you hooked. Do you really need to add to the number of things you already crave? If you do indulge and wind up derailed, tell yourself you are only one meal or one walk away from getting back on track. The sooner you get back on track, the better. The only thing worth missing is your health.

Show Me the Money

I hear all the time how it costs more money to eat healthy than not to. When it comes to organic foods, I agree. At a minimum, I try to at least get organic spinach, blueberries, and dairy. If you can't afford organic, it is still better to wash your non-organic berries and grab some nuts than it is to have a candy bar! Frozen fruits, vegetables, eggs, oatmeal, and beans are also cheap. Save money by buying fewer processed packaged food items and more fresh and frozen fruits and vegetables! It's true that fast food can be dirt cheap and more enticing. I know because I make the rounds myself. I usually wind up driving through when it comes to back-to-back sports and school activities. Yet I pay attention to what I order and give my children one carb option, not three. For me, it's a salad with protein and some nuts from the stash in my purse. I do not consider fast food a destination location. I also do not consider this perfect parenting. However, this is learning how to balance options instead of blindly overdoing it. In chapter 7, there are ideas for how to balance your children's day by starting off with a decent breakfast, healthy lunch, and a real food snack so a fast-food stop for dinner here and there does not have to derail their progress.

I will never forget when one of the young health care providers I worked with gushed in announcing she had been to a certain fast-food establishment three times that day because it was "half-price" day. She had driven through for breakfast, lunch, and dinner, getting a shake at every pass along with her meal. Out of the goodness of her heart, she also picked up fries for one of her grandparents. The grandparent was hypoglycemic and could no longer have the coveted shakes, so the granddaughter chose fries for her instead, *three times that day*. It is a blessing to see anyone thinking of a grandparent once a day, let alone three times! However, the $1.99 saved on all of those half-priced fries and shakes is not even going to put a dent in this family's future health care costs.

Make Your Move

The balanced scales of justice are a great reminder to balance out movement and food intake today. Telling yourself you will one day exercise and lose weight when things finally calm down is a pipe dream. If you think a stress-free life is the prerequisite for weight loss, you may be surprised.

SUMMER IN THE CITY

Living the dream. After sixteen years of both active and reserve time with the Navy, my husband and I were able to share the same address. I joined him in the San Francisco Bay Area for the summer while he participated in his internship program with a company that later hired him upon completion of his graduate degree. It was the first and last time in my adult life that I was completely stress-free. I remember walking the Golden Gate Bridge with no phone or beeper (dating myself here). It was glorious! I worked out every day, walked the city, saw the sites, made friends along the way, and had fantastic dinners every night. There was only one problem with this blissful existence. Even though I blasted through major calories with fun activities, exercising all day and eating healthy most of the time, *I actually gained weight.* My husband's summer internship graciously provided lots of wining and dining, and we partook in all of it. One late-night free dinner gourmand experience after another took its toll. The realization hit that I certainly couldn't blame the weight gain on stress or a lack of exercise! All roads led to the late-night overconsumption of rich foods as the culprit. I remember a joke we played on each other during this time. My husband and I would put out each other's running shoes the night before, suggesting we needed to run it all off the next morning. We were still naïve enough to believe you could out-exercise a bad diet.

You may ask what this has to do with your stress and weight management. First, if you wait for the perfect time and situation to occur in life where you are stress-free, it will likely be in vain; it is most likely not going to happen.

If it does, it may not have the outcome you predict. A lot of empty nesters gain weight because they are going out and overdoing it at dinner every night. Second, whether or not you are fortunate enough to have a stress-free existence, you need to ask, Are you eating your way through a city? Takeout, fast food, and pizza most nights are going to give the same results. If you are running around on vacation, you may be active and burn it off, but it's typically not going to be enough.

Unfortunately, most people are sitting at a desk all day and then rushing around with kids in traffic after work. Progress will only be made once the realization hits that food is the final frontier. Managing diet is the only way to lose weight. Most people have no idea of how to make this switch in a culture that supports supersizing everything, but where there is a will, there is a way. As you are inspired to do it, turn to the appendix to execute the way. I am at fast-food establishments more often than I like to admit, with both boys in club soccer, school sports, and a myriad of other activities. However, I follow the charts in the appendix and have a salad, a vegetable with a protein, and some healthy fat. The same goes for vacations, late-night dinners, and conferences. Whether it is gourmet or fast food, I eat according to plan.

THE OTHERS

In the beginning, you can always find excuses not to get started with healthy eating or exercising. However, once you are hooked, you will find reasons to make it happen. Until then, a few potential roadblocks may need to be cleared.

One of my clients loved to walk but did not feel comfortable doing it alone. Because of this, she did not walk in her neighborhood. She also did not like the idea of mall walking because she wanted to be outside. She thought walking her neighborhood might be a good idea, but the minute she drove home after dropping the kids off, she felt compelled to go inside to straighten out the house. The walk never happened. I suggested she drive to two nearby parks she liked that were popular and well traveled. She listened and checked them out but decided she still liked her neighborhood better. She finally started walking in her neighborhood, but it took her driving to two different parks to come to this conclusion. The walk would not have happened had she not looked at the other options and decided her best bet was right under her nose. That's okay! Although she still walked alone, she ran into friends and neighbors and enjoyed that aspect. The point is sometimes you just have to take action to wind up right where you started.

Another client did not feel comfortable exercising at home with her husband because she felt he was judging her. Either she wasn't doing enough or she was overdoing it. Although other issues needed to be addressed, the end result was her not exercising. Once this was pointed out to her, she decided the gym was the only way to go, and they worked on the rest.

In both cases, these women had to figure out a way to make things work. Since the end result was both of these women exercising, both answers were correct. If they had not exercised because of someone else (present or not), they would have allowed someone else or their perception of the situation to control them. The same thing happens with food choices. I hear spouses say, "Now that you are on a new diet, should you really be eating certain foods?" There are snide comments like, "Here we go again," insinuating since other diets have failed, this one will meet the same fate. Of course this leads to anger, which is understandable. There is only one problem. Now the anger is controlling you. The next thing you know, you are taking out your anger on a tub of Ben and Jerry's. Is the person inciting you really the one you want in charge of your body? I have news for you. They are not the ones who will be sitting in your place at the doctor's office. Something will eventually work, but I can also guarantee nothing will work if you quit trying. I often remember a quote my father-in-law sent my sons when they were starting a new school, "Difficult beginnings do not have to mean bad endings" (Bill Bower).

Movement

There's a saying: if you don't use it, you lose it. Part of finding balance is moving your body in all different planes of motion. You may tend to do the same type of movements, overusing your muscles in one direction while underutilizing them in another. The result may be muscle imbalances or injuries. When I teach exercise classes, I teach total body resistance training. I recommend a class or an app that works your total body, emphasizing low weights with high reps. Include a warm-up in the beginning and gentle flexibility stretching at the end. I have included a sample movement schedule.

The joy of the Lord is your strength.

—*Nehemiah 8:10 (NIV)*

MOVEMENT GUIDE

DAILY MOVEMENT

- Move all day.
- No more than thirty minutes of sitting at a time.
- Pace when you are on the phone.
- Take the stairs to a bathroom on the next floor.
- Use a pedometer app.
- Try walking meetings.

BEGINNER CARDIO

Three to four days per week: thirty to forty-five minutes of steady state aerobic cardio (yes, walking counts, at a brisk pace)—bike, swim, jog, Zumba, and so on.

- Almost every piece of equipment at the gym shows aerobic and anaerobic heart rate zones. Stay aerobic.
- Yoga does not count as cardio. Boxing and kickboxing count as interval cardio.
- Review the "Make Your Move" section in week three for best exercises for your body type.

RESISTANCE TRAINING

Minimum two days per week: Incorporate some type of total body resistance training. Look for high repetition with low-weight workouts. If you enjoy yoga or Pilates, this can count as your third resistance day.

Flexibility

You don't have to take a yoga class, but you do need to stretch daily. Do a quick stretch after workouts. At the end of the day, hit all your muscle groups. Stretching can lower cortisol levels. Some studies show that stretching can also increase melatonin levels that help with sleep. There is also some evidence that total body stretching may assist in the prevention of atherosclerosis (plaque buildup in arteries).

Circuit Training

Combine resistance and interval training. Try a bike with small weights and do high reps of different arm movements while in aerobic zone pedaling. Then put the weights down and sprint on the bike for one minute. Repeat this until you finish your upper body workout on the bike. Then do core work, lower body moves, and stretch. (This is an efficient way to be done with both resistance and cardio interval training.) If you do intense circuit training, keep your other cardio days easy. You don't want intensity more than three days a week.

Intermediate Cardio

Intermediate. Two to three days per week, thirty to forty-five minutes: Warm up. Proceed to your aerobic zone. After 5 minutes, work up to the lower end of your anaerobic zone and maintain for thirty seconds to one minute. Repeat until time is up. Only incorporate interval training if you have a cardio base. (A cardio base means you can sustain an aerobic heart rate for thirty to forty-five minutes four days a week.)

Sample Week

Monday: thirty minutes interval on bike

Tuesday: resistance training (low weights with high reps)

Wednesday: thirty minutes interval on elliptical

Thursday: resistance training (Pilates)

Friday: thirty minutes interval (choice: swim, walk/jog, box)

Saturday: resistance training (power yoga)

Sunday: active rest (More to come on this in chapter 5. For now, go for a walk with your family or try a family bike ride. Recreate your energy.)

Advanced Cardio

Advanced. Thirty minutes: Warm up. Proceed to your aerobic zone. After three minutes, spend one minute in the lower end of your anaerobic zone and maintain for thirty seconds to one minute. Repeat until time is up. When that gets easy, after two minutes in your aerobic zone, work up to the lower end of your anaerobic zone for thirty seconds to one minute. Repeat. (Max three days per week.)

Take a Stand

Don't Hide Your Lamp Under a Bushel

Humility is not about being less than who God created you to be. It is about being the person you are meant to be—no more and no less. We need you to be that person. However, sometimes we are guilty of taking our gifts and distorting their value. Beauty is a great example of this. When it comes to weight, some women manipulate it because they are ashamed of their beauty, punishing themselves for something from their past. Beauty is a gift from God, and so is femininity. I know women who have gained weight because they do not want male attention or they do not want to stick out. I honestly think some would be skinny if this was the way to get lost in a crowd.

In almost every case, this is either because of a past injustice (abuse) or it is something they feel the need to punish themselves over (not forgiving themselves). Unhealthy choices are made out of fear or a feeling of unworthiness. Many are single or married women who by this world's standards are successful, yet they feel safer when they can fit in and get lost in the crowd. We all feel safer when we do not stand out in any area of our lives. However, beauty can never be blamed for someone else's wrong choices or our own. There are many examples of how beauty was used in the Bible to further God's plan. God must love beauty. It is one of the many good things He has blessed us with. What we do with it or how it has been exploited, twisted, or abused is a different matter. Beauty does not have to equal vanity or a lack of modesty, just like money does not have to equal greed. Besides, it brings a much-needed smile to our hearts. Why do you think God created beauty in the first place?

You are altogether beautiful, my darling; there is no flaw in you.

—Song of Solomon 4:7 (NIV)

Not living up to your full potential, in whatever category that may be, affects everyone you encounter to a greater or lesser degree. When you live in victory, you are setting an example encouraging everyone else around you to do the same. They may only know it is possible because of you!

Who knows if you haven't come to the kingdom for such a time as this?

—*Esther 4:14 (WEB)*

Love Your Neighbor

Just like we have to learn how to ask for help, we also have to learn how to say no. One of the reasons we get off balance is we struggle with setting limits. Even Jesus set limits with His time, based on what the Father was calling Him to do. We need to do the same, or we will miss out on what the Father is calling us to do.

Within Mark, chapter 1, there are two examples of Jesus setting limits. First, Jesus heals Simon's mother-in-law of a debilitating illness, so completely that she was able to immediately begin serving Him as if she were never sick. Afterward, the whole city gathered at their doorstep, hoping to be healed. Jesus healed many who were sick and drove out demons, but the next morning, He was gone. He went to a remote place in order to be alone with His Father. Simon later found Jesus and made sure Jesus was well aware that "everyone was looking for Him." In other words, "Where were you?" People were still seeking Him out. Yet Jesus considered time with His Father as nonnegotiable. If Jesus considered time with His Father as a top priority, I doubt you or I could come up with something better. Although His time on earth was short and there were still plenty of people waiting to be healed, time with His Father, typically in the morning, was nonnegotiable. You also have a limited time on earth, with plenty of people to help. Only God can answer the question of who and how since He is the one who has equipped you for this work.

The second way Jesus showed us how to set limits through these verses was His reply to Simon after Simon told Jesus everyone was looking for Him.

> He said to them, "Let us go into the nearby towns, that I may preach there also. For that is why I have come."
>
> —Mark 1:38 (MEV)

Although people were still seeking Jesus out in order to be healed, it was time for Him to move on. Most of us would have wallowed in guilt leaving behind anyone asking for help, let alone a whole city. Yet this was not His choice. He came to do His Father's will. Even Jesus knew He could not be in two places at once. This should pretty much sum it up for us also. If the time hasn't come already, a time will come where you will have to decide to do what God is calling you to do even if it disappoints someone else. This is why pleasing people cannot take priority over following Jesus. However, if you stop doing what others are asking of you, you may get accused of not acting like a Christian. This determination is between you and Christ and no one else.

As you start making healthier choices, others may get defensive about their own behavior. They take it personally and sometimes subconsciously try to sabotage your efforts. Unfortunately, since others have failed at weight loss in the past, watching someone else succeed brings up a lot of their unresolved issues. You can easily be blamed for their insecurities. You may question yourself and once again get caught up in everyone else instead of focusing on God. This is just another form of distraction keeping you from doing your Father's will. Many people fall into this bottomless pit of people pleasing instead of relying on what God is calling them to do. There will always be people and things demanding your time and energy. This does not mean you are supposed to ignore what God is calling you to do. Just like any other area of your life where you want success, you have to prioritize. Focusing on everyone else instead of God wastes time. Setting limits, even if it means not signing up for every single event at work or school or not always eating junk, may separate you, but this is not a bad thing. You have been set apart to make a difference in people's lives.

> *"Before I formed you in the womb I knew you, before you were born,*
> *I set you apart."*
>
> —*Jeremiah 1:5 (NIV)*

One way Christians are called to make a difference is by fighting injustices. You glorify God when you fight injustice, whether justice is served on your watch or not, because you are loving your neighbor in the process. For many, this can also be a path to healing.

CHANGE YOUR LIFE

Week Four: Justice

And the heavens proclaim his righteousness, for he is a God of justice.
—*Psalm 50:6 (NIV)*

For Your Soul

Do you trust God? If you struggle with justice being served, ask the Holy Spirit to illuminate God's Word for you specifically in this area.

In your nightly letter to God (NLG), ask yourself:

Is there a sin or unhealthy behavior you are justifying because in your mind justice has not been served?

Is there someone you need to forgive? Put Jesus in between you and that person.

Is there someone you resent because you think they have a better life than you?

Are you acting justly toward others? Are you acting justly toward yourself?

Do you need a heart transplant in order to take God at His Word? Ask for one.

Thou shalt not covet thy neighbor's skinny jeans.

Forgive as the Lord has forgiven you.

Love yourself as much as you love your neighbor.

Say yes to God so you can say no to the things hindering His plan for your life.

Is there an injustice you have been set apart for in order to make a difference for your neighbor and/or to help you heal?

For Your Body

Thank God for what your body is able to do today.

Nurture your nature.

Eat the amount you need of high-quality real food. Keep low quality to a minimum.

When it comes to sugar, you are not missing anything.

Stress-free does not equal fat-free.

Use the Movement Guide to plan workouts for your whole body.

Balance your food intake with your movement for optimal energy.

Perseverance

But those who hope in the Lord will renew their strength.
They will soar on wings like eagles; they will run and not grow weary,
they will walk and not be faint.

—Isaiah 40:31 (NIV)

When I taught FAITH VS. WEIGHT at the YMCA, I told participants they would get a full refund if they could come up with a legitimate excuse not to exercise after going through this program. Five years, a different location, and many classes later, no one has been able to come up with any excuse, not even the lawyers. How was I able to pull this off? I had help. In order to get people to stop making excuses regarding exercise, I gave them examples of real people who had plenty of real excuses not to exercise, but did it anyway. These people inspired me on the days I felt like giving up. We all have those days, months, and sometimes even years when we feel like throwing in the towel. Although these common people with an uncommon perseverance may not have one million Twitter followers, their example has already had an eternal impact. They may not be famous by earthly standards, but who knows what crown awaits them in heaven?

Blessed is the one who perseveres under trial because, having stood the test, that person will receive the crown of life that the Lord has promised to those who love him.

—James 1:12 (NIV)

While I was at the YMCA, I became a certified trainer for Livestrong, a program designed to help cancer survivors resume exercise, or in some cases, begin. I was exposed to one life after another picking up the pieces and starting all over again. If you think you have a good excuse not to exercise, what about those people? It would be one thing if they just had cancer, but rarely does someone just have cancer. There are complications from surgeries, ports, medications, and comorbidities. My clients also shared the heartache of their children struggling to understand their disease as well as their spouses trying to cope with it. Many held down jobs in the midst of trying to put their lives back together. There were days they felt nauseous, dizzy, weak, scared, and tired. They also shared how hard it was to look in the mirror and not recognize themselves. Yet they got in their car, drove to the gym, walked through the doors, and got busy. I had never seen such a group of fighters. They were fighting for their lives.

At the time, I was happily serving a variety of clients at the YMCA and had just completed my first half marathon, finishing in the top 25 percent. Life was good! Within two weeks, I was trying to figure out how to use a motorized cart at the grocery store since that was the year I broke my leg skiing at Whistler. Once I returned to the States, my doctor told me my leg would never regain its original strength. There were no guarantees I'd run again. Because my exercise options were limited, I needed to get creative. As long as I only used my arms and a flotation device, I was able to get my cardio exercise by swimming. In order to get in and out of the pool, I needed a chair lift and staff to help me use it. Although I did not wind up at a rehab pool, others used the same facility at designated times of the day for similar reasons.

In the pool to the right of me was someone I will call Dave. He had MS. He looked to be in his early forties, with severely limited leg mobility. Dave would drive to the gym and patiently get out of his car, get into his motorized chair, motor to the locker room, get ready to swim, motor to the pool, and then get in the pool, with no assistance from the chair lift. Before I barely had a chance to say hello, Dave was always asking how far I had come along with my recovery. I can't tell you what a humbling experience this was for me. I would later see him at church every Sunday with his wife and children. He would talk to me about the portion of the ride he was training for as a participant of the MS 150, the largest bike fundraising event of its kind in North America. Even though he had limited leg mobility, he was able to ride, and ride he did.

To the left lane was someone I will call Glen. He was in his thirties and was paralyzed from the waist down. I don't remember ever seeing Glen without a smile. He was always cheerful with a genuine concern for others. Glen would joke with me about my arm stroke, telling me how strong I was getting. Meanwhile, I marveled at his arm strength getting in and out of the pool, once again without the use of his legs or the chair lift.

Then there was Barbara. Barbara was in her seventies and still competed in a variety of sports. She was completely able bodied, just a little slower than her prime. This woman never stopped moving. I used to joke with her, telling her the reason she was not married was because she would have to rob the cradle in order to find someone who could keep up! She never focused on her aches and pains, only on moving herself and others forward.

And the Crown Goes To ...

That same year, our beloved Aunt Carol went on a mission trip to Rancho Sordo Mundo, a Christian school for the deaf, near Ensenada, Mexico. This was not her first year serving as part of a team escorting her local church's high school youth group. She had just turned seventy-six. On what she thought would be her last day of the trip, before heading back to the States, Carol and another chaperone were hit by a semi-tractor. Although the physicians did all they could, Carol had a below-the-knee amputation on her right leg. They salvaged what they could of her left foot. Instead of allowing this tragedy to cripple her emotionally, she forgave the driver and did not prosecute. She knew he had a young family and wanted him to be there for his children.

After enduring twelve surgeries, rehab, and hyperbaric treatments, see if you can guess where she went. Mexico, of course, on another mission trip—the first chance she got. I saw her at my in-laws' fiftieth wedding anniversary a few years back, and she had more vim and vigor than most people half her age. As a matter of fact, she looked amazing, which was shocking after all she had been through. Besides walking her dog, traveling with her church choir, and a dizzying array of volunteer commitments, somewhere in there I heard swimming. Even at eighty-two, it's hard to keep up with Aunt Carol. She recently returned from a trip to the Holy Land, as one of the oldest in her group of forty-two travelers, enjoying every site—while walking the entire time.

What excuse do you have not to exercise? I understand when clients do not feel like exercising, but perseverance is not based on a feeling. Among those who persevere, there is enduring love, joy, peace, patience, kindness, goodness, faithfulness, gentleness, and self-control, all fruits of the Holy Spirit. I would also add forgiveness.

"The righteous *keep moving* forward, and those with clean hands become stronger and stronger." —Job 17:9 (NLT)

Love the Lord Your God

Though the fig tree should not blossom And there be no fruit on the vines, Though the yield of the olive should fail And the fields produce no food, Though the flock should be cut off from the fold And there be no cattle in the stalls. Yet I will exult in the LORD, I will rejoice in the God of my salvation. The Lord GOD is my strength, And He has made my feet like hinds' feet, And makes me walk on my high places.

—Habakkuk 3:17–19 (NASB)

We all struggle to go the distance. It is easy to get discouraged by the many things that seem to work against us. You may be dealing with a serious family issue, health concern, divorce, or a troubled teen. Whatever the case, you are not alone.

Habakkuk knew he was not going it alone either. Because of this, he knew he could rejoice in the midst of his suffering. Although throughout the Old Testament the "high places" were locations used for idol worship, Habakkuk's reference to the "high places" was a state of being in the presence of the glory of God. This is where the Lord lifted him up. The "hinds' feet" represented swift access. You also have the opportunity to go swiftly to the high places as you rejoice in the Lord. When you lift the Lord up in worship, you are also being lifted up into the presence of His glory. Since perseverance is overcoming challenging situations that are unresolved over long periods of time, you would be wise to take advantage of visiting the high places. There is no vacation spot that is going to give you a better view of your circumstances or recharge your battery. The high places are as close as you get to heaven on earth.

WORSHIP WHILE YOU WAIT

Worshipping God is different from giving Him a laundry list of complaints. Worshipping God is meditating on His glory. It is acknowledging He is the King of kings and the Lord of lords.

Is anything too hard for the LORD?

—Genesis 18:14 (NIV)

Besides unconfessed sin, the reason we do not see more of God's power is that we do not recognize His glory. If you need help with this, look up at the night sky, watch the sun rise, read the Psalms, and listen to worship music. Another form of worship is meditating on God's Word by memorizing it. Although plenty of research shows the benefit of meditation for your health, when you meditate on God's Word by memorizing scripture, you are now taking meditation to a heavenly level. Worshipping God gets you out of your head and into His magnificent glory. Although that alone is worth the price of admission, when you recognize God's glory, you cannot help but also recognize His power.

God has spoken once, Twice I have heard this: That power belongs to God.

—Psalm 62:11 (NKJV)

VICTORY

The horse is made ready for the day of battle, but the victory belongs to the LORD.

—Proverbs 21:31 (NRSV)

I hate to break this to you, but in this case, you and I are the horse. We have to do the best we can to get ready for the battle. This is called perseverance. I often find people just hoping to get by with the bare minimum. Could this be one of the reasons we are not seeing many victories? Having extremely low expectations and putting in minimally haphazard efforts on an inconsistent basis is surviving, not thriving. This applies to both your faith and your weight. Instead, do the best you can, whenever you can, and you will be able to do more than you think you can. This is what I learned from my heroes.

The Bible is filled with victories that show you what God can do in and through you. However, many victories do not happen overnight, nor do they happen without your participation. If they happened overnight, we wouldn't realize they were victories. Your participation is where perseverance comes in. Perseverance is consistently doing your part, while acknowledging His glory. "The victory belongs to the Lord."

GOD'S POWER

> *And his incomparably great power for us who believe. That power is the same as the mighty strength he exerted when he raised Christ from the dead and seated him at his right hand in the heavenly realms.*
>
> *—Ephesians 1:19–20 (NIV)*

When the woman discussed in Mark, chapter 5, touched the hem of Jesus's cloak, Jesus felt power leave Him. If you are a follower of the Lord Jesus Christ, you also have access to God's unlimited power. It is the same power that raised Christ from the dead. However, sometimes even the faithful limit God's power by forgetting or not acknowledging His glory.

> *Yes, again and again they tempted God, And limited the Holy One of Israel. They did not remember His power: The day when He redeemed them from the enemy.*
>
> *—Psalm 78:41–42 (NKJV)*

If you plan on persevering, stop underestimating God's power. As mere mortals, you and I may not be able to fully comprehend it. However, you can go to the high places daily to be reminded of His glory. A failure to acknowledge God's glory is the reason I believe so many never see His power. They never see the victory they long for.

STRENGTH FOR THE BATTLE

> *This is what the LORD says to you: "Do not be afraid or discouraged of this vast army. For the battle is not yours, but God's."*
>
> *—2 Chronicles 20:15 (NIV)*

Not only is the victory not yours, neither is the battle! I see many people fighting internal battles all of the time. Lies strategically placed by Satan. Can I get an amen? Could it be that you are not winning the battle because you are the one fighting it? Your job is to go to Jesus and have Him fight on your behalf. It's His battle, not yours. It doesn't matter how big the battle is. If you are not responsible for the victory or the battle, then what exactly are you responsible for? Someone has to make the horse ready for the battle. Do not over or underestimate this effort. When it comes to your faith, you need to spend time with God before the battles come so that you are confident in your offense as well as your defense. When it comes to your health, you need to do your best and let God take care of the rest. Our role is to get battle ready. Many people take better care of their pets than they do themselves! It's time to love, feed, and train yourself for victory. Paralysis by analysis is guaranteed to keep you by the side of the pool. You are not in control of the outcome. Stop obsessing over the outcome (scale, etc.). This will make you into an invalid. Instead, put your energy into doing your best and leave the battle to the one who likes to show off His glory. He is undefeated.

FAITH WHILE YOU WAIT

Lead me in your truth, and teach me, for you are the God of my salvation; for you I wait all day long.

—*Psalm 25:5 (NRSV)*

Depending on how much weight you have to lose, it may seem like the wait is not worth it. Since the time will pass whether you are making progress or not, you might as well use the wait to your advantage. Remember the two-year gym example. Most of us think we are doing something wrong when we have to wait because it can be uncomfortable. Yet the Bible frequently mentions waiting on the Lord. Sometimes the whole purpose of the wait is for us to learn how to wait. In life, there is never a perfect time, and you will always be waiting for something, so you might as well get good at it. Waiting is the norm, not the exception. Many people think there is nothing they can do while they wait, but that's just not the case. You can visit the high places for the power to persevere as you continue to get the horse ready for battle.

Who comforts us in all our affliction, that we may be able to comfort those who are in any affliction, through the comfort with which we ourselves are comforted by God.

—2 Corinthians 1:4 (WEB)

You can also comfort others as they wait. Waiting may not be what you had in mind, but it is a great teacher. It does not mean that God has forgotten you. Waiting teaches you that you are not in control of the timing or the outcome. God is. The only one who can deliver you from your battle in the nick of time is the one who created time. His timing is better. You may be looking for a solution over here when He already has the problem solved over there. Not everything is intended for everybody, or maybe it is just not intended for you yet, but His intentions for you are better. If you pay attention, it gives you a chance to see His glory, not yours, but you have to persevere in order to see it. That often means waiting, but His glory is worth it. As the Lord comforts you while you wait, you will learn how to comfort others.

WORTH THE WAIT

God is in the midst of her, she shall not be moved; God shall help her, just at the break of dawn.

—Psalm 46:5 (NKJV)

Little did I know the first six months after I broke my leg would be a walk in the park compared to the rest of 2013. As I was learning how to walk without a limp, I tore one of my rotator cuffs. The doctors concluded it started, and was further aggravated, when I went up and down the stairs in my house, favoring one shoulder over another because of my leg. Next was an overuse injury in my good leg since it took the brunt of my weight. On the heels of that injury, completely unrelated, came pancreatitis and finally gallbladder surgery, all within twelve months. By the end of the year, I was feeling pretty banged up. Although none of my health issues were debilitating, we weren't always clear as to what was going on with me medically. Before my doctors were able to figure out my gallbladder was the root cause of the problem with my pancreas, I had many nights of burning pain in my abdomen. It took a few months and thousands of dollars' worth of tests (thank God for insurance) before the doctors were able to diagnose the root cause. The first ultrasound showed a pancreatic head mass that was later downgraded to "pancreatic head fullness." Something to celebrate! This didn't sound great, but it was way better than the alternative.

My doctors had always suspected it was my gallbladder, but since I did not have gallstones, it was not obvious. The final exam showed my gallbladder was only operating at 30 percent efficiency. My mother had to have her gallbladder removed in her thirties, so in retrospect, this came as no surprise. Even though I lived a healthy life, as far as we could tell, this was not something I could prevent. The timing of my gallbladder puttering out within months after I broke my leg and tore my rotator cuff was less than ideal. Because of the gallbladder issue triggering pancreatitis, leaving me with burning acid, I had to start taking a daily dose of 60 mg of proton pump inhibitors (PPIs) to ease the pain.

In the meantime, like every parent, I tried to put my best foot forward for my kids. Between medical tests, physical therapy, and needing to get things done at a much slower pace, my husband had to pick up the slack, which also made things more difficult for everyone involved. He wound up having to have surgery that same year for a double hernia. We had the same surgeon!

I kept trying my hardest to jump back into activities, but the reality was that it was just not happening at the pace I wanted it to happen. I was on God's timeline, not mine. Pride and impatience were a constant battle. Ironically, the location where I broke my leg at Whistler is called Ego Bowl. What a wonderful reminder when it came to keeping my pride in check!

Besides having to rearrange certain parts of my life at certain times to keep my duties as a mom afloat, the hardest part of that year was not the broken leg, torn rotator cuff, pancreatitis, or gallbladder surgery. The hardest part was waiting four months for a diagnosis as I was continuing to decline. As a parent, it was hard not to worry since I was in pain and had less and less energy for my family. Thankfully, it turned out that waiting for the diagnosis was actually more stressful than the actual diagnosis. However, while I was waiting, I had a decision to make: did I trust God, whatever the outcome, or not?

> *Elijah came near to all the people and said, "How long will you hesitate between two opinions? If the Lord is God, follow Him; but if Baal, follow him." But the people did not answer him a word.*
>
> *—1 Kings 18:21 (NASB)*

In this case, God is the one who is waiting. I believe in some cases we are involved in creating our own delays. In my case, I finally realized the Lord was waiting for me. I could either waste time worrying or redeem time by worshipping, and only one of these options leads to victory in Christ. During this season, it was revealed to me there were things on the inside holding me back in my walk with the Lord. Decisions I had made in recent years needed to be reprioritized. Certain strongholds had to be let go of, almost surgically removed. I really don't think it was an accident that my accident happened on Ego Bowl. I doubt I would have noticed any of this had I not been forced to step back and wait. As a matter of fact, I am pretty sure I would not have noticed it at all. Maybe I wasn't just waiting after all.

Once I figured out I needed to spend time in the high places worshipping the Lord, things started falling into the right places. I don't want to give the impression that the Lord beats us down until we submit. However, I do want to convey my sincere belief that He wanted my undivided attention, and He knew I needed to be brought to the end of myself before I was willing to give it. This may have been tough love, but it pales in comparison with love everlasting. Sometimes we need to wait because we would not get the message any other way. Two years later, my family and I were born again.

> *The fear of the LORD is the beginning of wisdom, and knowledge of the Holy One is understanding.*
>
> *—Proverbs 9:10 (NIV)*

Moving On

We all have things we need to let go of in order to move on. An injury, disease, or disability may preclude you from doing certain activities temporarily or for the rest of your life, but I am not talking about activities. I am talking about fear. I believe the reason the invalid never made it into the pool of Bethesda was fear. Even though he was so close to his miracle, because of fear, he gave up before he even started. What are you afraid of? Ask Jehovah Raphe (the Lord your Healer) to expose it and heal you. Ask Him to help you let go once and for all of the fear holding you back at the cellular level. Then boldly take the next step.

After recovering from my challenging medical year, I had a lingering fear of skiing. Although I had ran, biked, swam, jumped, climbed, and danced before the Lord plenty of times, I had not skied. My entire family skis Whistler ever year, and every year my youngest son asked if I would ski again. I was physically able, but I was afraid. It didn't matter if I ever skied again, but the fear bothered me, because I felt it was holding me back in other areas. In my case, I had to go to another type of high place to conquer it.

I knew at some point Whistler and I would have another rendezvous because that mountain represented a year of struggle. It didn't just remind me of a broken leg; it reminded me of that entire year. I had no intention of skiing it, but it was time to look down it for once instead of constantly looking up at it. Mountains seem smaller once you are at the top. So I rode the Whistler Peak 2 Peak gondola to Blackomb Mountain and back, taking in the fantastic vistas from a glass-bottom gondola. The Peak 2 Peak is one of the world's longest continuous, unsupported, highest lift systems of its kind, with a (free) span of 1.88 miles. Just riding it is a leap of faith. Its highest point is 1,427 feet above the ground. I would not have done it had my boys' ski instructor not suggested we all meet at the top of Whistler for lunch.

We can't always go back, but sometimes going back helps us to release and move on. Chatting over lunch, our boys' ski instructor asked me why I didn't ski. Once I told her about the accident, she told me that my fear was locked in at the cellular level, and there was a need for healing. I never said I was afraid, but it was obvious. This was not the conversation I expected to have with a ski instructor on top of a mountain over a salmon salad, but Deb Hillary was not your typical ski instructor. Because of the years she invested training her own boys, as of this writing, they are among the top skiers in the world.

When I think about releasing fear at the cellular level, I think about the one who created our cells. The one who created our cells is the only one who can heal them. He may use others to help do this, if they or we are willing to be His hands and His feet, but in many cases, we have to take the first step. I wouldn't have had the conversation on the mountain that day if I hadn't stepped on the gondola, and it wouldn't have happened that day if she hadn't brought it up in the first place. Either way, I had to take the first step. Our physical healing can occur like the invalid at the pool at Bethesda, but just like the invalid, there may still be something holding us back. Lots of people are walking around who are physically intact that have gaping holes inside of them. Because of this, the invalid sat next to his miracle for thirty-eight years.

Before I knew it, the day came for my rendezvous with Whistler. One year after talking with Deb, I decided to ski the same mountain where I had broken my leg five years prior. I had no desire to take up skiing again. I just wanted to conquer that mountain! After several false starts, Deb coached me through my fears, and I finally relaxed enough to enjoy the breathtaking views. As I was skiing, I started noticing details about the other skiers. There were people of all ages and stages, including a group of instructors leading blind skiers down the mountain. Although the blind skiers could not see where they were going, they did not allow fear to keep them from moving forward. On that day on that mountain, we were all moving forward together. You may not be able to see where you are going either, but God does. What is your mountain? In order to persevere, ask God to help you overcome your fear one step at a time.

For we walk by faith, not by sight.

—*2 Corinthians 5:7 (NRSV)*

Change Your Brain

You don't find your future spouse, get married, have a baby, and send kids off to college overnight. Perseverance is working on one thing at a time. Even God doesn't expect you to make all of those changes overnight. Why expect this from yourself when it comes to a lifetime of habits and then get discouraged when you don't change overnight?

THE DREAM

"The dream was always running ahead of me. To catch up, to live for a moment in unison, was the miracle" (Anaïs Nin). No matter how good you are at organizing and planning ahead, I guarantee, if it hasn't happened already, there will be something you will hope for with all of your heart that will not happen on your time frame. It may not happen at all, no matter what you do to try to make it happen. If you trust God, then not getting what you hoped for is actually better than getting what you had hoped for.

> Take delight in the LORD, and he will give you the desires of your heart.
>
> —Psalm 37:4 (NIV)

This verse is not about you actualizing your dreams but about Him actualizing His glory. When you take delight in the Lord, His vision for your life becomes your dreams. In this case, the fulfillment of your dreams will just be a matter of time. Ask Him to help you long for what He longs for. Like many people, I have dreamed dreams that were realized ten, twenty, or even thirty years later. For example, when I was a child, I dreamt someday I would live in a house with a mother and father who loved each other. Thirty years after I dreamt it, I now live in a house where the mother and father love each other, with God as their center. That would be my husband and I. The point is "not now" does not equal "not ever." It may actually equal something better, but you won't find out unless you persevere. I also thank God for the dreams He did not allow to come to fruition more than the ones that did!

"My soul with satisfaction of all wants, because God's gifts put man's best dreams to shame" (Elizabeth Barrett Browning, "Sonnets from the Portuguese 26").

What Are You Waiting For?

The devil wants you in despair while you are waiting. This will be your time of greatest temptation, and nothing will bring you down faster than despair. Losing weight takes time. You should also expect to be tempted just as Jesus was in the desert. In the past, it may have been with one too many desserts for one too many years, leading to diabetes. Maybe it was with one glass of wine at a time … as you decided to numb yourself through an unhappy marriage. This is not waiting on the Lord. Going forward, you will be tempted to take shortcuts. It could be in taking diet pills, shots, hormones, above what is medically necessary, or overdoing supplements instead of investing the time in doing your part while trusting the Lord to do His. Shortcuts on the front end typically equal greater delays on the back end.

Like Habakkuk, instead of dwelling in despair, we need to focus on God's capabilities instead of our current inabilities. The waiting room is your date with destiny. Your ability to decide on what to focus your energy on while you wait is a gift from God. What you choose to do with this gift influences your destiny. You will find plenty of examples of waiting in the Bible, some handled in better ways than others. More often than not, the waiting is meant to teach you something. Why not learn the lesson sooner rather than later?

The Waiting Room

The waiting room can be a location like a doctor's office. You may be there for yourself, your child, your spouse, or another loved one. It can be waiting for test results, a new drug protocol, the end of chemo, or your eyebrows to grow back after chemo. It can be waiting to have a child, or waiting on a rebellious teenager to turn to God. It can be waiting to get married or for a divorce to be finalized. Sometimes waiting seems like a lifetime if you or someone in your family is living with a chronic condition/addiction. While you are waiting, there are usually times when things seem to be getting worse instead of better. In some cases, the options seem to be dwindling, just like they were for Habakkuk. You can choose to worry, which usually results in visiting the closest vending machine, or you can rejoice in the Lord. The fastest way to get to the high places is by listening to praise and worship music.

But I will sing of Your power; Yes, I will sing aloud of Your mercy in the morning; for You have been my defense And refuge in the day of my trouble.

—*Psalm 59:16 (NKJV)*

Eat for Energy

IN IT TO WIN IT

How is that some people keep the weight off while others put it back on? First, you must believe it is possible to lose weight *and* maintain weight loss. Many believe in the first half of this statement but not the second. This is because once they achieve their ideal weight, they return to eating with a vengeance. Significantly more calories are consumed once people are off their diets with the additional handicap of less muscle mass. This process repeats itself with every crash diet. The only way to avoid this is to maintain something you can live with. This is why the FAITH VS. WEIGHT diet is a lifestyle. Many clients tell me this is just the way they eat now, because they are happy with it.

Crash dieting is one of the fastest ways to lose muscle mass. Resistance training is imperative in regaining lost muscle mass from pregnancies, aging, and crash diets. You don't need to bulk up, but you do need to work your muscles enough to wake up your metabolism. Sprint intervals as part of your cardio helps with fat loss, but you still need to bring some muscle back into the equation by adding resistance training.

When challenges arise, be prepared. If you are succeeding in sticking with one dessert a day at home but get off track when you are away from home, surrounded by sugar for long periods, you need a backup plan. Long meetings with doughnuts/cookies or a lingering client dinner with unlimited desserts, especially when you have already had your one dessert, can be painful. As a backup plan, I carry teabags in my purse. You can almost always get hot water. This works if you wind up getting stuck with at a lot of late-night dinners or never-ending meetings. Also make sure you have a hundred-calorie bag of nuts on hand. Even if you have already had your nuts for the day, it is always—I repeat, *always*—better to have one hundred calories of a satiety food like nuts than "just a bite" of something you know is going to derail you. I would much rather have an additional hundred-calorie bag of nuts than overdo it by consuming hundreds of calories of cookies. Remember prudence: what is the most likely outcome?

I Will Survive

I have four theories regarding reasons people regain weight after a restrictive diet:

1.   Sugar addiction
2.   Emotional eating
3.   Binge eating
4.   Decrease in activity level without a decrease in calories

1) Sugar Addiction

Some people can still be friends after a break up, and some cannot. It is the same with sugar. This may be linked to serotonin and dopamine levels or a full moon. Whatever the case, instead of beating yourself up and feeling like a loser, realize this is probably no more than a biochemical situation. Some researchers believe if addictive tendencies run in your family, sugar can also be a problem. Since this is the case with almost every other person, it is hard to tell. If sugar is an issue, you have two options.

Option 1

Once people get their blood sugar under control, it is much easier to have a small amount of sugar as a dessert at the end of the day. This is how most cultures have dessert around the world. However, if you are highly sugar sensitive, you will most likely not be able to have any amount of any type of dessert with sugar in it. You need to be more selective. To determine whether or not this applies to you, stick to this plan for three days in a row. Make sure you are not including artificial sweeteners, sugary drinks, dessert samples, or starchy carbs during the day. In the evening when you would normally have dessert, try one hundred calories of plain (no fruit or nuts) 70 to 80 percent dark chocolate. This is an experiment to see if you can satiate your palate with a dessert that contains more fat than sugar, rather than eating desserts with ingredients that cause you to want more. I prefer Alter Eco black truffles, plain dark chocolate made with a small amount of coconut oil that curbs hunger. One is enough. Black truffles are not flavored. You can branch out later to see if you can enjoy other flavors without overdoing it, but for now, look at this as if you were conducting an experiment. By isolating one flavor (chocolate), we are avoiding others that may hyperstimulate your palate because they contain ingredients, either sweet or salty, causing you to want more.

Instead of finding variety in your dessert, you can find variety in what you have with it. For example, if you love mint, enjoy Moroccan mint or peppermint tea. If you love cherry, have your truffle with a black cherry herbal tea. Make sure you are not buying teas with sugar added. Read the label.

If you are following the plan, but you are still having a problem with sugar portion control, then it is time to try varying your starchy carbohydrate timing. Perhaps you should time your starchy carb after dessert to make it easier for you to stop at just one dark chocolate during dessert. Having your starchy carb with dinner, since it is before your dessert, may make it more difficult for you to control your sugar intake. Even though the starchy carbs listed on this plan are slow carbs, any starchy carbs before dessert may make your blood sugar fluctuate. Experiment with timing.

Controlling your glycemic response makes it much easier for you not to overdo sugar. However, the way to change behavior is not solely physiological, it is also psychological. When my clients tell themselves, "I can have my treat tonight," it helps them say no to the junk they encounter all day. Again, this is not the Last Supper. If you can choose one hundred calories today, then you can choose it again tomorrow, the next day, and the day after that.

The idea of not totally cutting out dessert is based on the theory of "harm reduction" used with addicts. Harm reduction is used when someone who is addicted wants to quit, or at least cut down, but cannot. They need intervention. This is the reason why, when, what, and how to eat are described in this book. By eating high-quality foods early and often, you minimize blood sugar crashes that trigger mood swings and lead to wanting to grab whatever happens to be in front of you. If you have tried these suggestions but are still unable to stop eating before half the bag of single-serve dark chocolates are gone, or if chocolate is just not your thing, then I suggest option 2.

Option 2

Is it time to stop eating sugar? If this puts you in panic mode, you may very well be highly motivated to try option 1, in all earnest, one more time. If that still doesn't work, just say no. Saying no to sugar is not something that should make you sad! Remember this program is about fullness of life. Just like alcohol, sugar is not worth God's glory. If you are like the Israelites wandering in the dessert for forty years, maybe you have been on this mountain long enough.

The first few days are the hardest, but it does get easier! For some, sugar is more physiologically addicting than for others. This is why you need a few days to detox. Remember the breakup analogy that some can be friends after a split, and some cannot. As is the case with all unhealthy relationships, there is life after sugar. Some people move on to popcorn and nuts. Try no sugar for three days and see how you feel. The irony of the situation is many celebrities spend thousands of dollars on trainers only to come to the same conclusion. Consider the money you just saved!

Of course, most people do not choose to give up sugar as a permanent fix. This is the reason this book first suggests you learn how to incorporate sugar in small amounts as a dessert, instead of omitting sugar. If you went straight to no sugar but still had doubt in your mind as to whether or not you could figure out a way not to overdo it, you would wind up like most Americans. Because there is so much binging, most try to convince themselves that no sugar is the only answer. Then they wind up continuing to ricochet from binging to abstaining as the scale goes up, up, and away. This is why you want to give option 1 everything you've got before assuming you have no choice but option 2.

If no sugar is the right answer for you, you will know it. If not, don't give up on option 1. Find the small amount of dessert that works for you in the appropriate amount. Again, a higher proportion of fat to sugar usually helps. Whichever option you choose, you cannot do this alone. In all things, ask God for help. Whether you are asking for help in learning how to eat small amounts of sugar or avoid it all together, you will still need to ask for help.

The Mighty One, will save; He will rejoice over you with gladness. He will quiet you with His love, He will rejoice over you with singing.

—Zephaniah 3:17 (NKJV)

If you are ready to give sugar up, I recommend giving it up for three days. That's it. Then see how you feel. This is a decision point, where you either return to option 1 or continue with option 2. I also recommend you not tell anyone you are doing this, unless they are highly supportive, for those three days. You do not need to deal with negative fodder. In the beginning, every place you go will remind you of the one thing you are trying to give up. In this case, however, it is not your imagination, because sugar is everywhere! Just like the stories you hear of people drunk texting their ex, you will be irrationally convinced you can't live without it for three days, but you can. I promise! Like a bad breakup, you need to remember why you broke up in the first place. For some, this may mean multiple breakups until you are ready for the real thing. Many smokers try to quit several times before they finally quit. However, if you continually wind up overdoing sugar in your attempt to completely get rid of it, therein may lie your answer. It may be time to give option 1 another try.

Although this may sound like no help at all, if you are not sure where you belong, going through both experiences can help you choose the one most likely to work for you. How do I know this? I speak from experience.

In most cases, I do not eat the desserts everyone else eats. I am selective. Being selective allows me to not cut sugar out completely. This is a happy medium, especially if every time you decide to give up sugar, you wind up binging six out of seven days a week. However, the only way not to feel deprived is to find something that your mind still perceives as a treat that does not trigger a binge. This is how you master option 1. Get the idea? You may need to just keep trying until you can find something that feels like a treat but does not compel you to keep going. Just like some people may leave a job or career only to find out it was better than what they originally thought, you may have a similar experience. However, you may never know this unless you try both alternatives. There is no judgment either way.

2) Emotional Eating

He must increase, but I must decrease.

—John 3:30 (MEV)

If you invite more of Jesus into your life, your cravings for all other things will diminish. You will have fewer problems with emotional eating if you visit the high place daily. There are plenty of inspiring worship songs on iTunes, Pandora, and Spotify. When things spin into a catastrophe or "carb-tastrophe" mode, emotional eating emerges. When you are upset, worried, stressed out, or lonely, you are in the fight-or-flight mode. It's time to get out of your head. Taking a three-minute walk while listening to a worship song can make or break the rest of your day. Just like a child, sometimes we all have to redirect!

3) Binge Eating

Emotional eating may stop with an extra serving or two. Binge eating takes you into another territory. Although people do not like to talk about it, it happens more often than most realize. Like emotional eating, reaching for any substance other than what it is intended gets things out of whack. Food is meant to create energy, not self-medicate. Remember to pay attention to whether or not you relax when you eat—or eat to relax. If you are trying to eat to relax, you may never stop. Instead, take a deep breath and pray before you eat. This simple act helps relax you. It puts God in between you and whatever is causing you stress. It also puts God in between you and food. If this is a recurring issue, Christian counselors can help you get to the root of what is causing this behavior.

OBSERVATION VERSUS CONDEMNATION

Look at binge eating as if you are doing a scientific inquiry because that is what observation is. Leave the emotion out of it. Pay attention to the times during the day when you overindulge. You may also want to pay attention to whether or not you are being too restrictive at other times. Are you consuming enough calories throughout the day? If you skip breakfast every morning, it should come as no surprise when you binge at night. Skipping lunch and afternoon snacks almost always guarantee that you will overeat at dinnertime.

Make some non-emotional observations. Do you binge on certain foods at certain times? Write down how you feel before and after a binge. Have you cut out starchy carbs altogether and now you are inhaling the bread basket instead of having healthier starchy carbs in the evening as suggested on the plan? This is the reason there are no off-limits food categories on this plan. Instead of deeming a food category off-limits, find another food in the same category that you are able to limit. For example, in the sugar category, candy corns are something I can easily overeat, whereas I don't think I have ever had more than one black truffle. They are just too rich, and they are also made with real ingredients. Candy corns are what I like to call a virtual reality food. They are not really food. For me, corn syrup hyperstimulates my palate, causing the normal cues of satiety to malfunction. Most processed foods fall in this category.

In some cases, you may have a situation requiring medical intervention, whereas in others, you may just need to start eating single-ingredient real food. Real food comes as a single ingredient. An egg is just an egg. You are better off combining single-ingredient foods. You can mix an egg with vegetables, and now you have an omelet. You may also top it with some Parmesan cheese and olive oil. This is very different from going to a bakery and getting a piece of processed quiche. Know what you are eating.

Alcohol is like having concentrated sugar, which is another invitation for an all-out eating frenzy. Relaxed inhibitions accompanied with carbs, sugar, salt, and fat are never a good combination. Yes, I know Jesus drank wine, but He was not having it with all-you-can-eat nachos, chips, and queso or apricot-flavored brie and crackers. Besides, the alcohol content and entire process of making wine is very different now than it was then. If you can follow the FAITH VS. WEIGHT rule of "one or none" when it comes to alcohol and not overdo eating, you will be one of the few. Alcohol stimulates hunger. During week one, we discussed how food is meant to satisfy hunger, not create it. The real food God created satisfies your hunger. Processed foods with added salt, sugar, carbs, and bad fats do the opposite. We are not smarter than God in any area, especially this one! Throw alcohol in to the mix, and all bets are off.

There Is a Reason You Can't Eat Just One

Families with substance abuse or chemical dependency issues may have a tendency to overeat. Obese individuals' brains light up like a Christmas tree when they eat sugar. Do their brains light up because they are obese or is something causing their tendency toward obesity, stimulating their brains? I think it has more to do with the latter, having the physiological tendency in the first place. Just like alcoholics can't have one glass of wine, it is difficult for many people to have sugar without overdoing it. For those who are obese, it is harder. Regardless of whether or not the chicken or the egg came first, avoid foods that trigger binging. Get off of the train before it derails.

The Likely Suspects

Besides salt and bad fats, it is worth looking more in depth at these two other triggers:

Sugar. Even certain fruits can be dangerous ground. Low-glycemic berries (strawberries are a winner) and green apples (which for some, seem to be better than red) are a good choice. I also enjoy one half of a pink grapefruit. Stay away from dry fruits and tropical fruits other than yellow/green bananas. A banana is the same number of calories whether it is green or black. However, a green banana is mostly resistant starch, whereas a black banana is mostly sugar; think banana bread. Since resistant starch naturally blocks fat, greener is better. Other than fruit, most people do not realize that even milk can trigger sugar issues since it has a higher sugar content than most people realize. As for sweeteners, any sweetener that puts the taste of sugar in your mouth hyperstimulates your palate, causing you to crave more sweets. It doesn't matter if it is natural (stevia) or not. The only time I make an exception to this rule is for honey before a workout. See the eating timing and tips chart in the appendix. For dessert, stick with a higher fat-to-sugar ratio with real sugar. Fake sugars can make cravings worse. Keep dessert to one hundred calories.

Carbs. Pay attention to which carbs set off a binge. Since you are only having your starchy carbs at night, it will be easier to isolate this.

4) Decrease in Activity Level without a Decrease in Calories

You can start by cutting out unnecessary extras, but sooner or later you are going to have to move. If not, you will wind up with a small (or large) amount of weight creeping up over the years. As part of aging, your body composition goes from less muscle to more fat. Although menopause makes it worse, even eighty-year-olds have been shown to gain strength and increase muscle mass when introduced to resistance training. It is never too late. Start with resistance exercises along with a steady cardio base until you are ready to do interval cardio and take it up a notch. There is no reason you can't get stronger!

Faster Is Not Always Better

As a trainer, I have read hundreds of success stories. The most common theme is that each person starts somewhere, cuts back a little, changes a few eating habits at a time, has a setback, gets back on track, makes further corrections, has another setback, then recommits. Although this may not seem like the fastest way to lose weight, it is the most realistic for many. Most successful maintainers ease into losing the weight. This is the case of many hundred-pound-plus losers who have actually maintained their weight loss regardless of their approach. It did not happen overnight. Keep it simple. Pick one thing you can live with that will allow you to make progress. Once this is mastered, pick another. Perseverance is a process!

BORN AGAIN

If you have been born again and accepted the Lord Jesus Christ as your personal Savior, then you already know this does not mean you will never be tempted or backslide. The same applies to your health. Many health advocates are tempted and occasionally indulge in less than optimal choices. The difference is they have a firsthand knowledge of what happens if they continue down the wrong unhealthy path. So they get back on track. In your spiritual walk, when you falter, you also know better. You confess your sin and get back on track. The same applies to healthy eating. Just because you do not make 100 percent optimal eating choices 100 percent of the time does not mean you are not a healthy eater. This is not a pass/fail. This is a lifestyle. You are not reading this book to feel guilty; you are reading this book to get healthy. The decision you make for your next meal and activity can change your life.

Make Your Move

For the kingdom of God is not a matter of talk but of power.
—1 Corinthians 4:20 (NIV)

ACTIVE REST

We all have days we don't feel like doing a full workout. However, it is always better to keep moving forward in order to avoid slipping backward. Because of this, I am a huge advocate of active rest, which is basically a state of taking it easy while still being active. It may be a slow bike ride, a stroll, or chair aerobics if you have limited leg mobility. Active rest is not meant to be a hardcore workout. It is movement. Even if you do plan on working out five days a week, it can easily wind up only being three. If you don't have an active rest mind-set, your only other option when not working out is inactivity. One day of inactivity is not a problem. However, what typically happens is one day turns into a week before you know it. Then a week turns into a month. Cultures around the world are constantly moving at a more relaxed pace. This keeps joints lubricated, oxygen flowing, muscles engaged, and your heart and brain happy. As long as you are still moving, you are moving forward. Newton's first law of motion states, "A body at rest will remain at rest unless an outside force acts on it, and a body in motion at a constant velocity will remain in motion in a straight line unless acted upon by an outside force."

Take a Stand

Many people look at what they used to be able to do and stop dead in their tracks. Since they can't participate in whatever that was, they quit. This is not perseverance. If you cannot do something you used to love, fall in love with something else. Another path is open to you if you are open to finding it. You are called to do the best you can through all ages, stages, and phases of life. Whether you are dealing with an injury or recovering from a surgery, get the help you need in order to rehab while you are waiting to recover. Incorporate whatever gentle movement you can as soon as you can.

INJURIES/SURGERIES

When it comes to injuries or surgeries, it is not a foregone conclusion that you will gain weight. I had a senior client come to me who was scheduled to have multiple foot surgeries. She did not want to lose the momentum she had already built, so she decided to hire a trainer. I told her we were not only going to maintain her strength but would improve it wherever we could while she was waiting to get through her surgeries. And that is exactly what she accomplished while losing a few pounds in the process. She made it through like a champ and was a great inspiration to me.

Post-injury and post-surgery, you may want to stay in bed and pull the covers over your head. However, eventually you will get antsy. The problem comes when you are still not fully recovered. For many, this no-man's-land is more uncomfortable than the actual injury or surgery. Well-meaning friends may drop in with a meal or treat, and before you know it, you are eating lasagna and cookies all day. After the party is over, no one really wants to think about fitting back into their wardrobe. Increasing a size after medical issues is never a welcome experience. Even if you eat healthy, when you are less active, you will still lose some muscle and gain fat. That's because a decrease in muscle and activity causes things to shift. However, you can minimize this inevitability. One of the reasons it is so important to move whatever part of your body you can while recovering is to preserve or even gain muscle mass.

Movement combined with healthy eating will help you avoid excess pounds. This doesn't mean you have to do a marathon. It also does not mean you can't enjoy a treat. I actually encourage my recovering clients to still have some sort of treat they have picked out. It makes it easier to say no to the other junk that will come into the house. People seem to show up with lots of sugar when you are hurting. It is well meaning but also the last thing you need. Whether I am recovering from an injury or surgery or training for a 5K, my meals are the same as described on this plan. I may have one less carbohydrate at night if I am less active, but that's it. You don't have to gain weight while recovering. I didn't, and neither did my proactive client with her multiple foot surgeries. She actually lost weight.

Medical Conditions That May Cause Weight Gain

Maybe you have thyroid issues or are on medications that cause weight gain. As a YMCA Livestrong trainer, I worked with cancer survivors on steroids. As if having cancer is not challenging enough, dealing with excess weight gain is never easy. Telling yourself, "Since I am going to be fat anyway, I might as well just face-plant into a quart of ice cream," is not going to make things better. Once again, you will have two problems (or more) instead of the one you already have. Diabetes, high cholesterol, metabolic syndrome, and so on are not much fun either. Obviously medical conditions tend to leave people feeling uncomfortable. However, reaching for comfort foods is only going to make things worse. At some point, that extra ten to fifty pounds due to unhealthy choices will need to come off, or you may wind up with more health issues down the road. As far as I know, not many people want to extend their time as a patient! Eating poorly is not going to stop you from feeling poorly. It will only prolong the process and make things worse.

Cancer survivors and others going through a debilitating disease often have to deal with feeling unattractive. It is horrible when you are wondering if others are thinking about how awful you look. Focus your energy more on what God thinks. In Christ, you can emerge from these trials with a shimmering spirit. When people sense the light of Christ, they are drawn to it. There is nothing more beautiful. From a physical perspective, I have seen plenty of cancer survivors who ate healthy and exercised lose excess weight and get stronger. I am not a nutritionist or a physician, but it makes sense that as you take care of your body in one way, while you are waiting, you are helping other issues as well. The same goes with your spiritual health.

For the LORD does not see as man sees; for man looks at the outward appearance, but the LORD looks at the heart.

—1 Samuel 16:7 (NKJV)

When it comes to broken bones, sprains, and the like, take advantage of physical therapy or other recovery options available to you. Believing you have an influence over your recovery is a huge mental factor when it comes to weight management. Time and again, I hear people tell me about how they used to be in shape before a certain injury, and then one thing snowballed into another, and now they have a serious weight problem. This is sad to hear and more common than you think, but it is not a foregone conclusion.

Beyond healthy eating, physical therapy can be a major player when it comes to your healing process. Make therapy work for you instead of focusing your energy on feeling like a victim. Yes, it is a scheduling nightmare and one more thing to do. It can also be painful and frustrating. However, it can get you back to doing what you like or introduce you to a myriad of alternatives. Sticking with physical therapy has helped me get back in the game more than once. A good therapist can help you get your range of motion back while strengthening certain areas that will help you avoid future injuries or re-injuries due to weaknesses. You want to get three things from therapy: strength, flexibility, and balance. When you are strong, flexible, and have good balance, you have a much better chance of maintaining a healthy weight while avoiding future injuries. Don't shortcut therapy, even if it means just going to get the exercises.

Managed Care

If you are told from a medical perspective that you will have future limitations based on a diagnosis but feel the Holy Spirit is prompting you otherwise, ask God for direction. This also applies to the need for ongoing medications that may no longer be necessary. God is the only one who is capable of healing you. It's much better to focus on proving God right than to waste your time and energy trying to prove someone else wrong.

One of the most frequently prescribed medications, proton pump inhibitors (PPI), otherwise known as acid blockers, can be almost impossible to wean off of, even with medical care. Once my gallbladder was out, I was eventually able to get off of the high dose of PPIs I was on, but it was not easy. Even though the original problem was no longer there, my body had become dependent on these drugs. When I asked about decreasing my dose, I was told that I had to continue on the higher dose. Unfortunately, our health care system is not designed to help people decrease medications. Since I no longer had a gallbladder, the supposed root of my burning acid issues, I tried to stop taking the PPIs on my own but was unable to because of the pain. Although PPIs are not considered pain medication, I share this example since we clearly have problems as a nation weaning off of prescription medications, including pain meds, which is one of the reasons so many people are addicted to opioids. Just as people are prescribed necessary medication for pain, they also need to have a clear exit plan, decreasing dosage until the drug is no longer needed, but that's for another book.

Although I had to change doctors to obtain a *lower* dose prescription, by gradually decreasing the dose of the PPIs and tweaking my diet, I was finally able to stop taking them altogether. This was not an overnight process. My body slowly adjusted. The FAITH VS. WEIGHT diet is what has continued to keep me off of PPIs. On zero medications at my next annual physical, I was told I was above the ninety-fifth percentile in terms of my health. Had I not questioned the need to stay on a higher dose, I would still be on PPIs today. Not only are they expensive, they have long-term side effects, as do most drugs. That being said, because of the burning acid, I wouldn't have slept for the four-month period prior to having my gallbladder removed without them. I am thankful I had the option to take PPIs when I needed them. However, eventually with surgery and the appropriate lifestyle adjustments, they were no longer necessary. Listen to the Holy Spirit's prompting when it comes to your health. Are you currently taking pills for a condition that you could better manage by adopting a healthier lifestyle? This is not something to guess at. Find a doctor that will guide you in evaluating your current situation, and who is able to help you make the necessary transition to a lower dose, if appropriate. Almost all medications have side effects, with weight gain often being listed as one of the least offensive.

In all your ways submit to him, and he will make your paths straight.

—*Proverbs 3:6 (NIV)*

Love Your Neighbor

Helping others to persevere promotes longevity. Whether it is globally or locally, providing someone with a healthy meal, compassion, or a ride to church, studies show that volunteering is good for your mind and body. However, charity can go far beyond a meal or a ride. Jesus didn't just check off a to-do list when helping others. He loved. Sharing the love of Christ by praying with and for others, while serving as His hands and feet, mobilizes heaven on earth.

Sooner or later, we all need help in order to persevere, especially when we are also responsible for the care of others. No one realizes all of the things moms do until moms are unable to do them. Shopping, laundry, childcare, preparing meals, and driving kids to and from school along with their activities are further complicated when medical issues arise requiring frequent appointments, especially when Mom is unable to drive. When I broke my leg, my husband had a heavy travel schedule, so he was unable to pitch in during the week. My father-in-law, a retired rocket scientist, gave up a month of his life living on the central coast of California to care for our family in Texas. We couldn't have made it that first month without him! At the end of each long day of him cheerfully taking on whatever humble task needed to be done, this accomplished man would always ask if there was any other menial task he could help with before he went to bed! His servant heart readjusted my personal pride meter.

No stranger to charity, my mother-in-law, who is in her late seventies, decided to buy a car with wide doors so that she could drive the "old ladies" to church who didn't have a ride. She also serves by baking communion bread, participating in the hand bell choir, acting as a greeter, and volunteering on different committees. For years, she was involved in running the church's preschool. When my family was not able to be there, she was the one who helped with the births of both of our children. This barely covers the highlights. I don't have a better example of helping others persevere than these two folks.

Had they not actively taken care of their own health, they would not be able to continue to help both their older and younger neighbors persevere! Now in his early eighties, my father-in-law rides a stationary bike, enjoys running their local church's sound system, and chauffeurs his grandchildren to sporting and musical events. My mother-in-law keeps busy with all of the above, walks her neighborhood, drives her middle-school-aged grandchildren to soccer, and plays with the younger ones.

They have shown me that not only is it much better to be able to help others persevere than the alternative, it also keeps you young! Especially when you do it with love.

CHANGE YOUR LIFE

Week Five: Perseverance

Many are the afflictions of the righteous, But the Lord delivers him out of them all.

—*Psalm 34:19 (NKJV)*

For Your Soul

Are you now able to look at any excuses not to exercise in a new light?

What one step are you going to do this week to observe God's glory as you spend time in the high places? Which might work as a new daily habit?

- meditating/memorizing scripture
- reading the book of Psalms
- looking at the night sky or watching a sunrise or sunset while listening to worship music

Is anything holding you back in your walk with the Lord?

In your Bible, underline every verse in the Psalms that contains the word "power" in it.

Ask God to fight your battles. He is better at it.

Is fear affecting your ability to persevere? Conquer it in Jesus's name.

What are you waiting for? Ask Him to help you long for what He longs for you.

Are you surviving or persevering? Only one of them leads to victory.

Help your neighbor persevere. You just might get healthier in the process.

For Your Body

Identify whether or not your eating tends to fall in any of these categories: sugar addiction, emotional eating, binge eating, or a decrease in activity level without a decreases in calories.

Incorporate the suggestions recommended for your greatest problem area above and then move to the next one.

Work on observation instead of condemnation.

Are you committed to doing the best you can in order to persevere, whenever you can, physically preparing your body for the battle (eating healthy and exercising)?

What are you going to commit to do to get the "horse" ready regarding eating healthy?

What are you going to commit to do for exercise?

Incorporate active rest and move daily.

When recovering, take advantage of physical therapy and your doctor's recommendations. Then focus on the God who heals and not your problem.

Say no to excess "comfort foods." Excess weight is not a comfort when you are recovering.

Are there any medications you no longer need? Among other more serious complications from unnecessary long-term usage, weight gain is a common symptom. Check with your doctor to see if lifestyle changes can get you off of drugs. You may need to get a second opinion.

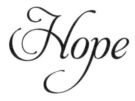

Hope

"For I know the plans I have for you," declares the LORD, "plans to prosper you and not to harm you, plans to give you hope and a future."

—*Jeremiah 29:11 (NIV)*

In 2017, the World Health Organization declared depression the number one illness worldwide, with anxiety as a close second. Breaking news tells us of celebrity suicides, with the overall suicide rate increasing dramatically. People who appear to have it all by this world's standards are in despair, including our youth. If you are having similar thoughts, please call 1-800-273-TALK.

Why are so many of us depressed? Symptoms of depression and anxiety are related to a lack of hope. It turns out that hope is one of the things you and I need most. Not surprisingly, excess weight has been linked to both anxiety and depression. Are we anxious or depressed because we are fat, or are we fat because we are anxious and depressed? It really doesn't matter. Whether your depression/anxiety is triggered by genetics; a biochemical imbalance; a stressful situation; or all of the above these mood disorders are highly treatable! There is hope!

Why have so many lost hope?

We are looking for comfort from a world unable to give it. Without God, there is no hope. If you get nothing else out of this chapter, please internalize the fact that feeling hopeless based on what this world has to offer is not only normal, it is biblical. Your hope is not in this world. Your hope is in the Lord. This chapter is about strengthening your hope in the Lord.

LET'S TALK

> *You, dear children, are from God and have overcome them, because the one who is in you is greater than the one who is in the world.*
>
> *—1 John 4:4 (NIV)*

Whatever the reason, people are still hesitant to talk about mental health as if they are the only one to ever go through these challenges (another lie of the devil, in order to isolate). You should know the numbers related to mental health diagnoses are even higher than those related to the obesity epidemic! So let's just get this out in the open! If you are suffering, please understand these four things:

Not only are you not alone, you are actually in the majority when it comes to diagnoses! The reason the numbers are so high is because many believe there is no hope, which is another lie from the devil. Your hope comes from the Lord.

"The one who is in you is greater" than any of your symptoms.

This is only a snapshot of your life, regardless of how long you have been suffering. It is not the whole movie, so please don't miss out on the best parts. Your future has not even started.

You are only one phone call or click away from getting the help you need. There are many trained licensed Christian counselors who are available for sessions by phone if you prefer not to physically go in for a consult. Check with your local Bible-believing church for references.

Since a lack of hope is a major symptom of depression, it's no wonder that many are convinced their situation is hopeless! Because of this circular logic, most people suffering from depression either do not get the help they need or rely solely on drugs to solve the problem. Rather, a combination of talk therapy with a licensed Christian counselor and medication are the most effective ways to initially combat these disorders. Because there is a strong tendency to want to be isolated when you are depressed, it is even more important that you do not delay, since this only makes things worse. Put this book down and get help today!

On Counseling

If you are waiting to feel more hopeful before you ask for help, you may be waiting a long time. Since depression, if ignored, can worsen over time, the sooner you get help, the better. Once you get help, you will wonder why you waited so long!

In order to have hope, we may also need to forgive others, God, and ourselves. At a minimum, most people need some type of support in order to forgive and be forgiven. This type of fellowship is fostered within a church community, as God intended it. However, in some cases, we need more. One-on-one sessions with trained professionals can help you identify and release strongholds that are holding you back with regard to your faith and your weight. If necessary, they can also refer you to specialists who deal with eating disorders. Surprisingly, the root cause of chronic overeating rarely has anything to do with food.

The View Only Gets Better

Come and hear, all you who fear God, And I will declare what He has done for my soul.

—Psalm 66:16 (NKJV)

You need to know that if you are depressed, whatever you are going through now is not permanent. This is just a snapshot compared to the rest of your life, both here on earth and beyond. It doesn't matter how old you are or what your current stage of life is. Your symptoms are not who you are. Your symptoms are not your destiny. He still "plans to give you a hope and a future"!

Although I did not have access to counseling as a child growing up in an abusive home, I spent two years in counseling as an adult. It was one of the best decisions I ever made. My only regret is that I didn't do it sooner. I was then able to release my past and embrace my future. That same freedom is available to you!

One Day at a Time

I remember being overweight, starting middle school, dealing (or rather not dealing) with depression after my parents' divorce. I was trying to find my new equilibrium while still caught in the middle of their various stages of anger. However, the timing of what occurred right after their divorce was the proverbial straw that broke the camel's back. I became the target of "mean girl" bullying from those who were previously my closest friends. From that day forward, school was no longer an escape from my home life. It became another lonely and fearful place. Later that same year, I was assaulted by three teenage boys, who I knew, during an attempted rape that I narrowly escaped. Although it was a miracle that I got away, this trifecta of events left me with a type of post-traumatic stress. Losing hope in family and friends, I eventually lost hope in myself. I cried myself to sleep many nights until I finally stopped crying. I was depressed.

Depression is an ominous feeling of being hyper-focused on an isolating despair that is based on a limited perception. We only see what we are currently focused on, and even that is narrow and gloomy. Hence the term *tunnel vision*. Because of this limited view, I did not see the prayer warriors who prayed for me as if their life depended on it, when it was actually mine that did. I also believe that because of their prayers, an angel of the Lord prompted my friend's older brother to walk around the corner at precisely the right time, sparing me from being raped by the three teenagers.

Prayer protected me in other ways as well. It took a few years, and things got worse before they got better. This is usually the time when people are tempted to give up on prayer, because they start wondering whether or not prayer is working. However, this is precisely the time prayer is needed the most. Because of the stalwart prayers of others, I finally realized my only hope was in the Lord. Depression is not a faith issue. It is a hope issue. This is why a lack of hope is listed as one of the main symptoms.

Storm Heaven

"For where two or three gather in my name, there am I with them."

—Matthew 18:20 (NIV)

In the meantime, ask others to storm heaven on your behalf. Ask them to pray for you. If you don't know anyone who can pray for you, or you do not feel comfortable asking, prayer request hotlines are available all over the country. If you do not know where to start, Prestonwood Baptist Church has online prayer requests available through their prayer ministry at preston-wood.org. Even better, set aside a time with friends to pray for each other over a weekly coffee. Bible studies at local churches are not only a great way to learn the Bible, they are also a wonderful way to meet some real prayer warriors. Do not underestimate the power of prayer; prayer moves mountains. Before you assume your situation is too hopeless for even prayer, where else do you plan on going for hope? Nobody is selling it. Drugs can make you feel better temporarily, until they make you feel worse, but even drugs do not give hope. Hope only comes from the Lord. So when should you give up on prayer? Do we pray only if our circumstances are improving or getting worse? Both.

Because he bends down to listen, I will pray as long as I have breath!

—Psalm 116:2 (NLT)

Even within healthy family situations with no additional trauma, the preteen through early adult years are difficult. Because of a lack of perspective along with hormones, the combined feeling of isolation and despair that can be experienced both at home and at school is often intensified. Yet these years are only a snapshot compared to the rest of your life. However, many people allow these years to wreak havoc for the rest of their lives. Your past does not need to ruin your future. The takeaway here is that this is true of depression regardless of what age it happens. Even if you have chronic depression, this is not who you are; these are symptoms you are experiencing. It is not a foregone conclusion that you will be depressed the rest of your life. Besides counseling, appropriate medication, and prayer, lifestyle can play a significant role, as we will cover later in this chapter. Just as your choices add up when it comes to your state of physical health, your choices also add up when it comes to your mental health. At the time of my depression, I felt completely hopeless, as if there was no point in going on, but my future had not even gotten started. Neither has yours!

I lift up my eyes to the mountains—where does my help come from?

—Psalm 121:1 (NIV)

Although some people can pinpoint a specific time when their hope was restored, mine has been more like climbing a mountain. I seem to get to a certain plateau until I learn what the Lord is trying to teach me before it is time to break camp and ascend to the next level. The Lord then calls me to even greater heights as my hope in Him surpasses previous stops along the way. There were certainly times I went down a few notches, but He lovingly lifted me up time and again. The view is amazing! It only keeps getting better. I can't wait to see what's next because my hope is in the Lord!

Whatever your current situation, Satan wants you to believe your current view is as good as it is gets. This is a lie. You still have mountains to climb, with some breathtaking views up ahead. Depression and anxiety, fueled by fear, are his specialties designed to try to keep you from your mountaintop experience. He wants you to believe there is no hope. Before you take this personally, this actually has nothing to do with you. It is God he is after. That is why the battle is the Lord's, not yours. So is the victory!

Are You Stuck?

Depression or anxiety may be a major factor hindering your weight-loss efforts. I have not taught a single class where these issues have not come up repeatedly. I have heard devastating stories of suffering from my clients concerning abuse and rape. However, there is also suffering associated with job loss, divorce, disease, wayward teenagers, multiple miscarriages, abortions, and childlessness. I pray with my clients. I have also cried and laughed with them. Yet the final answer never changes. If you need help, get it.

First, as in all things, ask Jesus to heal you, and second, pray for wise counsel. Then have others storm heaven on your behalf! Many people think they are too far gone or their problem is too mundane. Both are lies from the devil. As you go through this chapter, I want you to ask yourself if any of the areas mentioned are ones that may be holding you back. If so, it is time to get help. Here is the $64 million question/s when it comes to whether or not you need counseling. Are you stuck? How long have you been stuck? Are you able to get unstuck?

I didn't seek counseling until I realized I was stuck. Although I was successful by worldly measures, issues I had not dealt with from childhood were repeatedly sabotaging my happiness and relationships as an adult. I finally realized if my car was broken, I needed a mechanic. If my lights were out, I had to call the power company. So if I was emotionally stuck and living in my own created misery, I needed counseling! Most people do not like to admit to this or actually go through with it. It is kind of like physical therapy. It hurts in the beginning while you are first drudging up the injury, but the end goal is to get you back in the game, stronger than ever. Therapy is not meant to make you wallow in your most painful topic with no end in sight. It is meant to get to the root cause of the issue and then give you the practical tools to set your free. Where else can you voice your struggles to an understanding ear engaged in listening, not judging you, while also providing you with the tools necessary to move forward? Ask around for a trusted Christian counselor. Let me know if they have any other openings! So I can sign up again!

THE SHAME GAME

Then I heard a loud voice in heaven say: "Now have come the salvation and the power and the kingdom of our God, and the authority of his Messiah. For the accuser of our brothers and sisters, who accuses them before our God day and night, has been hurled down."

—Revelation 12:10 (NIV)

For many, obesity is one way of detaching from shame since it is a detachment from the needs of the body. Obviously, with the SAD (standard American diet), not everyone who has a weight issue is dealing with shame; yet in many cases, food is used as a coping mechanism for shame, anxiety, and depression. You may try to separate from your body because the "accuser" is still tormenting you over something that happened years ago. However, according to the verse above, the accuser has already been "hurled down." You don't need to listen to that garbage anymore. Nothing anyone has ever done to you or that you have done can separate you from God. You may be unique in a lot of areas but not this one. You have the same access to the all-encompassing love of the Lord Jesus Christ as anyone else. Human love cannot compare. You also have access to His power when it comes to taking care of your body. Whatever category you are in, staple the following verse to your brain. Repeat it. Absorb it. Feel free to insert not only your name but any family member or friend's name you are crying out to God for as well.

Neither height nor depth, nor anything else in all creation, will be able to separate [insert your name here] from the love of God that is in Christ Jesus our Lord.

—Romans 8:39 (NIV)

You Belong to the Lord

Don't you know that you yourselves are God's temple and that God's Spirit dwells in your midst? If anyone destroys God's temple, God will destroy that person; for God's temple is sacred, and you together are that temple.

—1 Corinthians 3:16–17 (NIV)

If you have been abused, you do not need to waste bitterness or wish for revenge. Why? Because the Lord says vengeance is His. You belong to the Lord. The reality is even if it were okay to take vengeance on another person, this is chump change compared to the wrath of God.

"I will execute great vengeance on them with wrathful rebukes; and they will know that I am the LORD when I lay My vengeance on them."

—Ezekiel 25:17 (NASB)

I wonder if the Lord takes vengeance out of our hands because He can do a much better job than we can. Our job is to forgive and to pray for the salvation of the person who has hurt us. As impossible as this may seem on your own, it is entirely possible with the Lord. When you forgive someone, you put God in between you and that person. It is no longer about them. Forgiveness reveals whether or not you trust God. When I am unable to forgive, I ask the Lord to supernaturally remove the anger from within me. It works. More importantly, it frees up energy for His glory.

Beloved, never avenge yourselves, but leave room for the wrath of God; for it is written, "Vengeance is mine, I will repay, says the Lord."

—Romans 12:19 (NRSV)

When someone acts outside of God's will, they are sinning against God first. You are not the only one who has been hurt. God has more than one reason to want vengeance. He hurts because of the sin against Him, and He hurts because of the sin against you. He has been hurt from every angle. However, even God knows who is behind the hurting. He is also hurt because the person doing the hurting has been led astray. This is why we need to pray for that person. They have been deceived by the father of lies, and they have to live with the consequences both now and in eternity.

> *Jesus said, "Father, forgive them, for they don't know what they are doing." Dividing his garments among them, they cast lots.*
>
> *—Luke 23:34 (WEB)*

Instead of putting the blame on the father of lies, where it belongs, sometimes we wind up being angry at or blaming/shaming ourselves. You see this a lot in spousal abuse and in adult victims of child abuse. Many abused women and adult victims of child abuse wind up believing it is their fault on some level because they are listening to the accuser. Since there is nothing worse than feeling out of control of a situation, we are looking for a way to bring some order to it. *Why did this happen? What did I do to cause or deserve this?* Many wind up blaming themselves.

> *Do not be overcome by evil, but overcome evil with good.*
>
> *—Romans 12:21 (NRSV)*

It is true these events represent chaos in our minds, but God is the only one who can bring order out of confusion. Blaming ourselves does not change the outcome. We do not have the power to go back in time, and even if we did, we are not the cause. We need to go forward, asking God for healing and peace. If we don't do this, we wind up with unhealthy behaviors later in life resulting from not releasing anger from past abuses. This affects everything from our health to our relationships. Diet alone is not going to fix this. Many people are unhealthy today because they are angry about something that happened yesterday. Suppressed anger wastes a tremendous amount of energy and is exhausting. If you are waiting for an apology or a relationship to be restored from someone who is either unable or unwilling, you could be waiting a really long time. Maybe even the rest of your life. How much of your future are you willing to waste on your past?

Submit yourselves, then, to God. Resist the devil, and he will flee from you.

—James 4:7 (NIV)

Past hurts seem to be like messages signed by the accuser, sealed in a bottle, floating out to sea, locked forever in time, never to be discovered or dealt with. How long ago did this happen? Is it still happening? Is it still happening in your head? Many people do not even realize they are sabotaging their health (and life) today because of a sin, either done to them or that they initiated, in some long-ago yesterday. The accuser then seizes this opportunity to trick you into thinking your legitimate need for healing can only be satisfied in illegitimate ways, so you stay stuck. Unfortunately, I see this like reruns from a bad soap opera over and over again with many new clients.

But as for you, you intended to harm me, but God intended it for good, in order to bring it about as it is this day, to save many lives.

—Genesis 50:20 (MEV)

If you want to get unstuck, you have to allow Jesus to heal you. Only you can do this! No one else can. If you are not allowing this to happen, then you are not allowing the Lord to use it for good. You cannot blame the person who hurt you for you not allowing God to heal you. You can't even blame God. He has been waiting to heal you. By allowing yourself to be healed, you now possess the potential to help heal many other lives in the process, starting with those closest to you. Not only does he "plan to give you a hope and a future," he even plans to restore your past in the process. That is, if you will let him.

So I will restore to you the years that the swarming locust has eaten.

—Joel 2:25 (NKJV)

Another reason many people struggle with a lack of hope and their weight is their unconfessed sin. This does not mean sin equals weight gain. However, it may mean that gnawing feeling in the pit of your stomach might lead you to start gnawing on food to try and alleviate the discomfort. You may have asked God for forgiveness and even stopped a particular sin. Did you remember to forgive yourself? Are you stuck because you cannot believe you are forgiven? Not believing God is able to forgive you is like not believing in God! If this is your struggle, it is just another lie from the accuser. If Satan can keep you feeling bad about your sin, he has a much better chance to get you to sin again. He wants your sin front and center. Instead, once you have confessed it before the one who knew no sin, you need to put your sin and the accuser behind you.

> *And Jesus answered and said to him, "Get behind Me, Satan! For it is written, 'You shall worship the Lord your God, and Him only you shall serve.'"*
>
> —*Luke 4:8 (NKJV)*

ANGER CAN MAKE YOU FAT

Whether you have unresolved anger with yourself, someone else, or God, anger can make you fat. Anger raises cortisol, which helps to store fat around your abdomen—the worst kind. Unresolved anger over long periods of time is toxic. Many people harbor unresolved anger for years and have turned it into a smoldering passive-aggressiveness. Anger not only affects mental health, possibly leading to depression and anxiety, but also causes physical stress on the body. Anger almost always leads to bad food and exercise choices. Do you typically associate a health nut with someone who is angry? Nope. Anger does not affect the other person's health. It affects your health. There is only one way out of unresolved anger. The answer is forgiveness.

> *Forgive as the Lord forgave you.*
>
> —*Colossians 3:13 (NIV)*

Forgiveness and peace were two of the main topics of Jesus's focus. They go hand and hand. When you are angry with someone, you typically do not trust that person, and there is no peace. Obviously, in some cases, you cannot trust a person who has not repented; however, you can still forgive them. You can still find peace. You don't need to wait on anyone else's actions for you to forgive them. You don't even need to wait until you feel ready, which is a day that may not come. Instead, all you need to do is ask Jesus to help you forgive. I cannot forgive on my own, and you cannot forgive on your own. This is why we need Jesus. Ask God to take away your anger, and He will.

Many people are not quite sure they want to let go of their anger. Too many are halfhearted when they ask for help to forgive. There is a part of them that thinks if they hold on to this anger, they are in some way controlling the situation. Subconscious thoughts may be similar to these: *I am still holding this person accountable. I am preventing this from happening again. I am preventing myself from getting hurt again.* Holding on to anger gives us some mistaken illusion we are in control. Since we suffered at the hands of another, we are searching for some way to make sense of this and want to control the situation. The problem is we were not and are not in control. Anger does not give you control. Anger produces misery, and misery leads to a lack of self-control, often triggering emotional overeating.

The only thing you have control over is whether or not you love the Lord your God with all your might. You do have control over that. Put your energy into serving the kingdom, making your own life and your neighbor's better. This is much better than wasting your energy on anger. Blaming other people for your unhappiness, even if they are responsible for miserable things, keeps them in charge. Is the person who hurt you really the one you want to keep in charge?

If you don't learn how to forgive others and yourself, you can easily fall into the deadly trap of anger at God. Many people walking around are angry with God. I can't speak for others, but I certainly have had my moments, as have many of my clients. I believe if you are honest with yourself, you may recognize some of these moments in your own life as well. Although not ideal, this is part of the human condition. The problem occurs when we feel we have either been let down or forgotten by God. Then we are not only angry but also disappointed.

It is easy to feel abandoned by God at some level if you feel like He has let you down, especially if you are still going through the motions of sitting in a pew every Sunday. If you feel you have been let down by God, you will not trust Him, and if you do not trust Him, it is impossible to have hope in Him. This is precisely why Satan wants you to believe you have been let down by God, just as he did with Eve. Instead, ask God to search your heart and purge it of anger and disappointment. In your nightly letter to God, ask Him to replace both with trust in Him. Forgiveness is not about trusting the other person. Forgiveness is about trusting God. If you want peace, you also need to learn how to forgive yourself. God has.

He has removed our sins as far from us as the east is from the west.

—Psalm 103:12 (NLT)

Anger will keep you fat, but more importantly, it creates a lack of trust, which obliterates hope. Your anger is not worth the glory of God!

RELEASED

For whoever does not love their brother and sister, whom they have seen, cannot love God, whom they have not seen.

—1 John 4:20 (NIV)

Forgiveness releases us from anger and regret, freeing us to love God and our neighbor. Almost twenty years after I had been bullied, the women who were involved started to feel regret. They were now mothers themselves. One of them called to apologize. The other had become friends with a family member of mine and asked my relative to convey the message to me that she had regret also. Yet, even if I had not forgiven, as long as they had repented before the Lord, my forgiveness would have been nice but not necessary for them. However, it would have been necessary for me. This is what people don't seem to get. When you forgive, you are the one who benefits the most. It frees you up to love the Lord and your neighbor. Not only is forgiveness good for your health, it is also one of the best opportunities you will have to share the Gospel.

*Jesus, standing up, saw her and said, "Woman, where are your ac-
cusers? Did no one condemn you?" She said, "No one, Lord." Jesus
said, "Neither do I condemn you. Go your way. From now on, sin no
more."*

—John 8:10–11 (WEB)

This Too Shall Pass

We all need to forgive in order to move on. One December, about seventeen
years ago, I was in the Navy and only able to get back to my hometown in
South Florida about once a year. I was a newlywed at the time, and my husband was joining me. It was our first married Christmas. Since my parents
were divorced, we had to split the visits, and for some reason this happened
to be the day we had planned to see my father. After dinner, I remembered
the decorated palm trees twinkling along the evening-lit waterways, and even
though there was no snow, the season was merry and bright. Thankfully, by
this point in my father's life, he had come to know the peace of Jesus. It was
not a moment too soon. After our goodbyes, my Dad stood by the door
waving until we were out of sight. I remember every detail of that night since
it was the last time I saw him alive.

*A person's days are determined; you have decreed the number of his
months and have set limits he cannot exceed.*

—Job 14:5 (NIV)

By the time my husband and I woke up the next morning, my father had
already gone to be with Jesus. Earlier that morning, a vehicle was backing
up, and the driver struck and killed my seventy-two-year-old father as he was
walking in a parking lot.

There were many decision points where I had to choose between anger and
forgiveness. I had Florida lawyers trying to convince me to sue everybody
and anybody, starting with the parking lot my father was killed in, claiming
there was inadequate lighting, to the driver. The woman who hit my father
started writing me letters. She was afraid of getting sued, but she was also

looking for something else. She needed to know she was forgiven. Just like the rest of us.

> *When they kept on questioning him, he straightened up and said to them, "Let any one of you who is without sin be the first to throw a stone at her."*
>
> —*John 8:7 (NIV)*

Although it was not easy, it was a perfect opportunity to share the light of Christ. I cannot say I was not angry or hurting. However, if I was going to call myself a Christian, I had to forgive, so I did. I made sure she knew this came from the love of Christ and not by my own doing. There were times I felt I put more energy into calming her down than I put into my own grieving, but I knew I had a role in releasing her flesh from the guilt she felt, for both of our sakes.

HE COMFORTS THOSE WHO MOURN

There were countless ways the Lord comforted me during this time, but here are some of the highlights. When the police gave me my father's wallet, I found a penny with a cross cut out in it. The coin and cross were completely undamaged. The other blessing was the fact that there were 364 days of that year where I was somewhere else. As mentioned, being in the military, I didn't make it home every Christmas. However, for that Christmas, The Lord gave me my father's last day on earth! During our visit, my father told me the Lord could take him at any time and that he felt completely at peace. I could actually sense it, neither of us knowing how imminent this was.

Finally, last year, I met a kind older man from our church. I had never met him before, but he said he liked to give people a small memento in order to share his faith. In my hand, he placed a penny with a cross cut out, identical to the one my father had on his body when he passed away. Of course the man had no idea what this meant to me, so I told him, especially since he had given me this gift on my father's birthday.

He will give a crown of beauty for ashes, a joyous blessing instead of mourning, festive praise instead of despair.

—*Isaiah 61:3 (NLT)*

Why bring up death in a book about weight loss? As a trainer, I have had countless clients tell me how the death of a parent or a loved one set off a massive weight gain. Heartbreak sends us reeling in all different directions, and food is just one of the things we use to cope. In many cases, we have to forgive and release. It is hard enough to deal with mourning, but when others are involved, there is often anger. Grieving is serious business and requires support. Grieving support groups provide an outlet that the rest of the world does not accommodate. Once you have sought help, the only way to get through times of mourning is to pay attention to all of the ways God is comforting you in the process. You are still here for a reason, and your family, friends, and church need you. If you need help with healing, forgiveness, or grieving, please seek it. Many people who try to "just get over it" wind up delaying the grieving process, only making it last longer.

PANIC ATTACKS

He leads me beside quiet waters, he refreshes my soul.

—*Psalm 23:2 (NIV)*

Anxiety can lead to panic attacks. A client has allowed me to share her story regarding panic attacks with the hope that her testimony will help others. This client had three children born with special needs, and the stress was overwhelming. Every night, she would wake up in a panic, convinced she was going to die from a heart attack. The ER staffs of all the local hospitals knew her by name.

This is her testimony …

> "After running to every hospital facility in town, I finally knew I was not in control of whether or not I lived or died. During a panic attack, I sat in a chair shaking all

over, with my heart pounding as if I were running a race in
the Olympics. I held onto the chair, and I repeatedly said,
"In the name of Jesus," and He comforted me. The attack
would then begin to subside, and I would function once
again. This time, without running to the hospital. Every
time after that, I grabbed a chair and sat when the panic
attacks started. I called on God. Eventually, I got better and
better. I no longer have these panic attacks. If I feel a small
panic attack trying to overwhelm me, I rebuke it (the devil),
and it disappears immediately. I have not had a panic attack
in years. Thank you, God. I truly believe without God's
intervention, I may have taken my life. Panic attacks are
so real they are truly not something you overcome without
help from God. Now, I am very peaceful and thankful that
He healed me from these attacks."

Years later, as this woman's trainer, I can testify that she lost seventy pounds
while exuding abundant joy. Confident and energetic, this is the last person
anyone would have ever assumed suffered from panic attacks.

Love the Lord Your God

*You who have shown me great and severe troubles, shall revive me
again and bring me up again from the depths of the earth. You shall
increase my greatness and comfort me on every side.*

—Psalm 71:20–21 (NKJV)

Anxiety levels are on the rise. As I write this, another school shooting is in
the news. This one happened thirty minutes from my childhood home. It's
hard to have hope in the midst of such unfathomable tragedy. Why does
God allow bad things to happen to good, innocent people? At first glance, it
seems like we live in chaos. We see lives and dreams cut short, leaving precious families and an entire nation crying out in mourning. The people who
commit these atrocities have bought into Satan's lie that they have no hope.

"The only saving faith is that which casts itself on God for life or death"
(Martin Luther).

When it comes to your faith, you will either cleave or leave. You will either
go deeper in your relationship with Jesus or abandon it. God is still on the
throne. He will show you comfort and mercy in unimaginable ways if you
let Him. Your job is to love and spread hope to those who are hurting in the
name of the Lord Jesus Christ, instead of wasting the time in fear and worry.

And can any of you by worrying add a single hour to your span of life?

—Matthew 6:27 (NRSV)

If Satan can't get you to outright deny God, he will do his best to render you
ineffective. Deceiving you into worry is one of his best tactics to manipulate
you. When you worry, you cannot spread hope, as the two cannot coexist. Satan wants you to believe your life is at the mercy of others, but your
Creator wants you to know you have security in Him alone.

Do not be afraid of those who kill the body but cannot kill the soul.

—Matthew 10:28 (NIV)

From Salvation to Sanctification

He was the greatest man among all the people of the East.

—Job 1:3 (NIV)

In one of the oldest books of the Bible dealing with hope, we meet Job. Job's story touches on all of life's toughest questions. Job was a good, upright man, obedient to the Lord. Satan dared God to take away everything (family, livelihood, and property) from Job because he was convinced once Job lost everything, he would curse God to His face. However, instead of cursing God, Job worshipped Him.

> *Naked I came from my mother's womb, and naked I will depart. The LORD gave and the LORD has taken away; may the name of the LORD be praised.*
>
> *—Job 1:21 (NIV)*

After Job was inflicted with boils, Job's wife finally said, "Are you still maintaining your integrity? Curse God and die!" However, Job still refused to curse God.

> *Shall we accept good from God, and not trouble.*
>
> *—Job 2:10 (NIV)*

When his friends heard how great Job's suffering was, they sat with him for seven days without speaking. Soon after, Job's friends assumed he must have done something terribly wrong to bring this calamity on himself. Yet Job still spoke as if God had the power to deliver Him.

> *I know that my redeemer lives, and that in the end he will stand on the earth.*
>
> *—Job 19:25 (NIV)*

In the meantime, Job answered his critics. He maintained he was not at fault. He also prayed for relief, but none came. You would think he would have long given up on God by now, but Job remained faithful.

I have not departed from the commandment of His lips; I have trea-
sured the words of His mouth more than my necessary food.

—Job 23:12 (NKJV)

Finally, the Lord came out of a storm to ultimately explain to Job there were
certain things he would never understand this side of heaven.

Where were you when I laid the earth's foundation? Tell me, if you
understand. Who marked off its dimensions? Surely you know! Who
stretched a measuring line across it? On what were its footings set, or
who laid its cornerstone—while the morning stars sang together and
all the angels shouted for joy?

—Job 38:4–7 (NIV)

On and on it went. The message here is that the faster we recognize we are
not God, and He is, the faster we will stop trying to figure out things we
are not meant to figure out, this side of heaven. If we can't even understand
how the existing things we see on a daily basis came into being, how can we
expect to understand how or why other things occur? Finally, Job put his
hand over his mouth in complete awe ...

I spoke once, but I have no answer, twice—but I will say no more.

— (Job 40:5 (NIV)

Job on Hope

Below are the five things about hope I learned from Job. They help me to
better understand not understanding.

I know that you can do all things; no purpose of yours can be thwarted.

—Job 42:2 (NIV)

No matter what anyone does to you or your family, God's plan for your life
and your children will not be thwarted. He knows the number of your days,
as well as what He is calling you and your children to complete in the time

allotted. He also has plans for you and your family in heaven. His view can be compared to one similar to a parent's, who can see the bigger picture a child is not quite able to wrap his head around yet.

Surely I spoke of things I did not understand.

—*Job 42:3 (NIV)*

Job realizes he has no idea of how God does things or why He allows certain things. None of us do. It is not necessary because we are not God. We must trust God and not our circumstances since we don't have the knowledge of the breadth or the depth of God's plan. There are many people who are unhappy because they are unable to accept that there are certain things they will never understand until they see Jesus. Spending time lamenting this reality during our short time on earth is futile.

Things too wonderful for me to know.

—*Job 42:3 (NIV)*

You are better off spending time in awe of the majesty of the glory of God and His creation. If you fail to do this, you will limit your view of His omnipotence. This leads you to assume He can't fix your problem or heal you. By assuming His reactions and responses should match yours instead of yours aspiring to be more like His, a storehouse of blessings is often left on the table. Job's hope remained in God even though He didn't know what God was going to do or how He was going to do it. Even if God did nothing, Job's hope still remained in the Lord.

Listen now, and I will speak; I will question you, and you shall answer me.

—*Job 42:4 (NIV)*

God listens. He wants you to talk to Him. You will have to answer to Him at some point. However, He also longs to reveal to you what you need to hear when you need to hear it. He wants you to flourish.

*My ears had heard of you but now my eyes have seen you. Therefore I
despise myself and repent in dust and ashes.*

—Job 42:5–6 (NIV)

For lack of a better word, you and I will be awestruck in the presence of
the Lord. In His presence, we will need to repent, because we will be overwhelmed by His purity. Yet He can still see our puny remnant of goodness.
Even though there were times Job felt forgotten and persecuted, he was
always esteemed in the eyes of the Lord. Because of this, the Lord healed Job
and blessed him with more children, seven sons and three daughters, while
twice restoring the number of livestock he previously owned.

*The LORD blessed the latter part of Job's life more than the former
part.*

—Job 42:12 (NIV)

Although Job was greatly rewarded, this was not the point of Job's suffering.
He was not suffering in order to get more stuff or replace a family he could
never replace. Job suffered for two reasons: first to glorify God, and second
to take his intimacy with God to the next level. This also prepared Job to
take on greater things.

The same applies to you. In order to do all God has called you to do for His
glory and your good, you will suffer. This happens for the same two reasons:
as an opportunity for God to manifest His glory and as an opportunity
for you to gain an insight you are unable to gain any other way. This also
prepares you to take on greater things for the kingdom. Suffering is a part of
your sanctification. When you are suffering, do not let go of God. Do not
let Him go until your trial restores your hope. Do not let Him go until He
blesses you. Better yet, do not let Him go, ever.

*Then the man said, "Let me go, for it is daybreak." But Jacob replied,
"I will not let you go unless you bless me."*

—Genesis 32:26 (NIV)

Change Your Brain

No, in all these things we are more than conquerors through him who loved us.

—Romans 8:37 (NIV)

Beyond medication and counseling, there are three key lifestyle factors you can significantly upgrade to dramatically improve your state of mind:

1. How you think
2. How you move
3. How you eat

There is good news on all three fronts! Each day we learn more about how our thoughts, movement, and food intake can influence our biochemistry, just like our biochemistry can influence our thoughts. When you think sad thoughts, you are cueing your body to put certain biochemical reactions in play. An example would be when you think of something upsetting, you start crying. The thought came first. Or you may have hormonal imbalances, common with many women going through menopause, and start crying because somebody looked at you funny. In this case, the biochemical reaction came first. Your physician needs to be involved to help diagnose your triggers in order to determine the type of help you need.

How You Think

Finally, brothers and sisters, whatever is true, whatever is noble, whatever is right, whatever is pure, whatever is lovely, whatever is admirable—if anything is excellent or praiseworthy—think about such things.

—Philippians 4:8 (NIV)

It is an assumption that people are born with healthy thought patterns. Even if someone grows up in a healthy, loving atmosphere, there are still biochemical factors at play, and they change. Also, we are born with original sin. Then there is Satan who is always on the prowl, constantly looking to poison people's thoughts.

So after getting medically evaluated, what can you do about this? What can you do to get your hopes up in general? The above verse tells you to "think about such things." This is probably one of the most compelling reasons to start your day off on a high note with the Lord. Even if you take precautions to focus on the right things, you are not in control of whatever else gets dumped on you during the day. It is imperative that you start off on a high note. As for the rest of your day, you have to be your own gatekeeper to the extent you can, especially if you are prone to anxiety or depression. Starting the day with negativity is only going to make things worse. The Bible continually talks about anxiety and fear because those are the two weapons most used against you, and the only way to successfully combat them is through the Word of God.

> *But whose delight is in the law of the LORD, and who meditates on his law day and night.*
>
> *—Psalm 1:2 (NIV)*

The only God-anointed way to control your thoughts is by meditating on His Word. This may sound like an overly simplified answer to all of your woes. That is because it is. Why make things more complicated than they need to be? Do we actually need to add more complication to our lives? Just for argument's sake, let's consider our alternatives. What else are you going to spend time meditating on? The news? Your career? Your finances? Your broken relationships? Just like Satan, all of these underdeliver, whereas God's Word does the opposite. God's Word promises to overdeliver.

> *He sent His word and healed them, And delivered them from their destructions.*
>
> *—Psalm 107:20 (NKJV)*

God Works

And we know that in all things God works for the good of those who love him, who have been called according to his purpose.

—Romans 8:28 (NIV)

Many who struggle with depression and anxiety second-guess whether or not God's plan for their life is good. Even if it seems as if nothing else is working, God is working for your good. Your road to recovery starts with believing God is working on your behalf. If you need help believing this, God already has someone picked out for you to talk to. It may be a family member, friend, pastor, or a health care provider. This is the first step toward your recovery. With God, there are no hopeless situations! Here are some other tips to get you started:

1. Use worship music. When King Saul was plagued by an evil spirit, he had David play his lyre. As a matter of fact, David was specifically brought there to play music. Music can bring relief to mood disorders.

Then relief would come to Saul; he would feel better, and the evil spirit would leave him.

—1 Samuel 16:23 (NIV)

2. Pick inspirational Bible verses. Put them on your calendar on your phone. Write them on note cards. Memorize them so they can uplift you during difficult times.

3. Listen or go to church. If you cannot attend regular church services, watch online. (Prestonwood.churchonline.org offers live streaming.) Eventually, it will be time to accept a friend's invitation to church. You can always sit in the back row! Being with people may be the last thing on your mind, but there is nothing like being lifted up by others singing praises to God. We are created to worship and have fellowship with others.

Anxiety in the heart of man causes depression, But a good word makes it glad.

—Proverbs 12:25 (NKJV)

Technology/Media

Peace I leave with you; my peace I give you. I do not give to you as the world gives. Do not let your hearts be troubled and do not be afraid.

—John 14:27 (NIV)

It is now the norm to be bombarded with negative messages from media, then sit all day at work, only to sit some more while stressed out in traffic, while eating junk. Is it any wonder why so many people are so miserable? There is something much more insidious going on with the constant barrage of negative information we take in that most people are oblivious to. We all know time spent in front of a screen makes you less active and more prone to weight gain. However, nobody really talks about what happens when we are bombarded with bad, often violent news from local and world sources real-time, from our televisions, computer screens, phones, and watches 24/7. On the milder side of tech, we are constantly being interrupted with another text or email request trying to fit one more thing into an already crammed schedule. Throw in some traffic with everyone texting at the same time, and you have the perfect storm. We live in an anxious world. If you happen to be a caretaker, you are also worried about those who are in your charge.

You would think after all of this we would recognize the need for a break. Instead of recharging by relaxing and unplugging during free time, we compare our life to everyone else's through the reliable source of social media. Everyone else seems to have it all together. Once we get through picking ourselves apart, we turn to entertainment to feel better, which is now mostly based on shock value. We either play a moral game of limbo, lowering the bar of what is left of our standards with each new television season, or we settle for binge watching one crime scene after another of people hurting themselves or others. Every person I know who watches these shows for fun later tells me they have nightmares. Doesn't sound like much fun to me!

Most people have no idea they are overeating because they are anxious, stressed, or depressed by their media choices. They also have no idea of how their media choices and 24/7 access to technology are instigating and aggravating these conditions. I believe one of the biggest reasons we "treat" ourselves with food is because we are looking to take the edge off of our self-induced anxiety. Carbohydrates increase serotonin and dopamine levels. Why do you think we call them comfort foods?

There is a correct amount and type of carbohydrate for each person, based on their activity level. Going below that number may cause as much anxiety as going above. Ever talk to a friend on a low-carb diet during her time of the month? Refined carbohydrates and sugars (which are also carbohydrates) give you the additional excitement of a blood sugar roller-coaster ride, leading to a crash that only exacerbates anxiety and the lows of depression. Combine this with watching the news and upsetting media, and you have a fat cocktail of toxic chemicals swirling around, contributing to the obesity epidemic. I often tell my clients I only watch the news when I am doing indoor exercise so I can expel the negative energy on a treadmill or bike, but only *after* I have spent time with the Lord.

We were not created to be bombarded with this world's problems all day every day, from the minute we wake up until our eyes glaze over and we pass out on the couch. Thank God He has not given us His job. This does not mean we should turn a blind eye. However, when it comes to protecting your mental health, if you don't do it nobody else will, and you can wind up getting so stressed out you are actually ineffective, in some cases paralyzed, when it comes to helping others.

> *We demolish arguments and every pretension that sets itself up against the knowledge of God, and we take captive every thought to make it obedient to Christ.*
>
> —*2 Corinthians 10:5 (NIV)*

Most people do not realize the toxic effect all of this noise has on their behavior. Eating ice cream while sitting on your couch hearing about yet another victim of a senseless crime does not have the same effect as a day trip to the spa. Your best food choices for raising serotonin levels (feel-good brain chemicals) are the carbohydrates recommended on the dinner/after dinner chart. Spoiler alert: it's not a quart of ice cream. A healthy diet and the right type of exercise, such as aerobic training like walking, calms a body down. In some cases, it has been shown to be as successful as medication when treating mild depression. Millions of dollars are being spent on studies to prove exercise should be available as a treatment for those suffering with mild depression. You can wait for those results or you can go for a walk and figure it out yourself. You can do a lot to keep yourself in the right frame of mind by starting your day with God and guarding yourself from unnecessary fodder second. Go for a walk instead.

Good Night

At night, to peacefully end the day, I read the notecards of past Bible verses I have memorized/meditated upon. This works much better than falling asleep to crime scenes. Instead, this is like greeting an old friend at the end of the day. It puts things in an eternal perspective, helping me to realize this too shall pass. For bigger issues, I write in my journal. This helps me to leave it all at the foot of the cross. It is fun to go back later and see how situations I once thought were insurmountable turn out to be chump change for the hand of God. You can start this tonight. As you find Bible verses that bring you peace, copy them on a notecard and place them by your bedside.

I have told you these things, so that in me you may have peace. In this world you will have trouble. But take heart! I have overcome the world.

—John 16:33 (NIV)

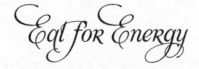

He who did not spare his own Son, but gave him up for us all—how
will he not also, along with him, graciously give us all things?

—Romans 8:32 (NIV)

How You Eat

Food and mood are inextricably linked. It's no accident He has graciously
given you all you need in the food He made to sustain a healthy mood.
However, we are all tempted by junk all day, every day. Bring on the chocolate-covered glazed doughnuts please! Food is easy, cheap, fast, and a great
distraction. It is all fun and games until somebody gets hurt with illnesses
like diabetes, heart disease, and excess weight! It also affects your state of
mind. In some cases, depending on what you are eating, food is the most
accessible drug around. Besides the problems associated with weight, it can
exacerbate depression and anxiety. Junk food does not alleviate your pain. It
makes depression and anxiety worse.

Besides exercise, real food makes a tremendous difference in keeping your
brain healthy. Omega-3s and coconut butter/oil substituted for other fats
seem to be high on the list for making your brain happy, while olive oil
seems to be good for both your brain and your heart. Vitamin D and the
B vitamins play a huge role when it comes to mood. It is worth checking
in with your doctor to have vitamin/mineral levels checked. What you eat
affects your mood more than you realize, since it can also influence your
hormone levels. Blaming all of your problems on hormones is not the answer
if you are mostly eating processed junk. Eat the rainbow instead. This is nonnegotiable when you are suffering from depression or anxiety. You cannot
expect your brain to perform happily when you don't put happy in it. Studies
show people are just plain happier when they eat more fruits and vegetables.

Do we really need more data on this one? Fish also seems to affect mood more positively than other proteins, most likely because of the omega-3.

You are your own chemistry set. How you run this chemistry experiment will determine the outcome. I notice a distinct difference in my mood after going a day of eating the SAD (standard American diet). I cannot sustain the SAD without feeling miserable physically and mentally. Most people do not even realize the SAD can cause physical and mental misery. Beyond enjoyment, you need to look at food as if it is a drug, because it is. This is no longer about not being able to fit into your skinny jeans; this is about feeling sluggish most of the time. Unfortunately, sluggish is a state of being for many people, and they don't even realize it. For many people, sluggish will eventually lead to sad. Eventually, we need larger or more frequent hits to keep ourselves up. This feeling is not a joyfully calm or peaceful existence. It is more of a hyper feeling of crash and burn.

Processed junk foods also exacerbate other diagnoses for adults and children, complicating issues that are already hard to diagnose and treat. Eating poorly is like throwing logs into the fireplace of inflammation. Food and mood may also affect other addictions. Most inpatient treatment centers for drug and alcohol advocate eating healthy; balanced meals at regular intervals help even out withdrawal symptoms.

Make Your Move

How You Move

Get outside in the sunlight every day for five to ten minutes at least three times a day! Sunlight makes a difference. If you are swamped, return phone calls as you walk outside the building. When it comes to your mood, the evidence in favor of being outside is overwhelmingly positive. If you are able to walk, bike, or enjoy another outdoor exercise, this is even better. Pets are also amazing companions for depression and binge eating disorders. They help you focus on something other than your symptoms. A light box may be something to explore if you are not in a part of the country where it's sunny.

Post-Partum

Years ago when I was a new mom, I had a dear friend who suffered from post-partum depression. Although she did not feel like going for a walk, she knew fresh air was good for her baby, so she agreed to walk with me. Every time we finished our stroll, she shared that she felt better. When people are depressed, exercise is the last thing on their mind. However, I tell my clients exercise is cheaper than Prozac! It is counterintuitive to exercise when you don't feel like getting out of bed, but the thing you often feel the least like doing may be exactly what you need to do to feel better! How do you find the energy to do this when you have no energy? Remind yourself ...

> *I can do all things through Christ, who strengthens me.*
>
> —*Philippians 4:13 (WEB)*

The mental benefits of exercise are the same or better than the physical benefits. When you are stuck, exercise can get you out of your head and beyond inertia. Isn't that part of the message of picking up your mat and walking?

Take a Stand

Many women suffer from anxiety and depression over life and death decisions they made years ago. It doesn't matter when it happened. Get the help you need today. These decisions no longer need to result in lingering pain. Is your ability to care for your health being affected by choices you made yesterday? Diet alone is not going to fix this problem. Another reason we struggle with caring for our health is unresolved grief that has not yet been placed at the foot of the cross. Your grief may be suspended in time. Maybe there was no ceremony or celebration of life to observe it or put it to rest.

In 1978, the first test-tube baby was born.

Since 1980, over a billion babies have been aborted worldwide.

The pain of not having a child while watching the world pass you by is gut-wrenching for many women. Infertility not only causes physical distress due to miscarriages but also emotional trauma. To increase the chance of conception, some women have decided on alternative solutions. IVF has become mainstream, yet just like when a natural pregnancy occurs, its success dwindles with the mother's age. That being said, we do see walking miracles every day because of IVF. Yet many other women suffer from a post-partum type of depression due to these procedures failing or from resulting miscarriages. Besides the resulting physical and emotional distress, this process does not always end up with a viable pregnancy. One of the side effects of IVF, regardless of whether or not it is successful, is weight gain. The heartache involved after multiple attempts is unbearable for some women.

Because the desire to have a child is so great, it does not always sink in that the possibility of additional fertilized eggs left over after IVF exists. Since a number of eggs have to be fertilized, there is no way of knowing which embryos will be successful or not. This means fertilized eggs that are not used. What happens to these embryos? They are either discarded or frozen. Women with frozen embryos may also be at a point in their lives where it is either not healthy to have another pregnancy or it is not financially viable, resulting in embryos left frozen year after year, until they are discarded. This is a hard thing to live with, especially if the woman is pro-life. There are some facilities that will accommodate donating eggs, but not all do. Most women are not focusing on this side of the story when first viewing IVF websites, seeing page after page of newborns. Conception has been and always will be a mystery.

Just as you do not know how the breath comes to the bones in the mother's womb, so you do not know the work of God, who makes everything.

—Ecclesiastes 11:5 (NRSV)

On the other hand, women who do have a successful procedure may wind up with multiple fetuses. Women who only wanted one child may wind up carrying two or more. These women have the option of selective reduction. Selective reduction is a medical term that basically means reducing the number of live fetuses. In some cases, selective reduction is recommended so that the stronger fetuses have a better chance at survival. Selective reduction can turn the joyous occasion of pregnancy, especially after so many years of waiting, into an occasion accompanied by unforeseeable regret.

Whatever the reason for an unplanned pregnancy, many women feel trapped. Women abort when they feel there is no hope for the future of their baby or for themselves when it comes to raising their child. This is another lie from the devil. Regardless of the reason, if you have had an abortion, you need to know God loves you. He always has, and He always will. If you are grieving from having an abortion, selective reduction, or discarding fertilized embryos, consider finding out about your local Rachel Ministry. These ministries break the bondage of guilt so healing can begin and women can move on with their lives, joyfully fulfilling whatever God is calling them (you) to do.

Now is your time of grief, but I will see you again and you will rejoice, and no one will take away your joy.

—John 16:22 (NIV)

Whether a mother is infertile or unable to care of her baby, adoption seems to cry out as the solution. There are thousands of children available to adopt through state agencies that need a home without having to wonder where their next meal is coming from or worse. Adoption gives a woman who is not able to conceive or carry a baby to term the chance to be a mother, while also giving another woman who is unable to care for her baby a place for her child to go. This gives three parties hope while also giving us a chance to care for the orphans in this world, which is much better than any of us living with the alternative.

If you are considering adoption, you do not need to go through this process alone. Chosen is the name of Prestonwood Baptist Church's ministry created to support and connect the community of people involved in the adoption experience at any point in their journey. Bible studies through Women's Ministry are also geared toward helping women heal after miscarriages and for those dealing with infertility. More churches are becoming aware of the need for this type of healing.

Love Your Neighbor

How You Love

What if you have a loved one dealing with anxiety and depression and you are the caregiver? Make sure you are taking care of yourself. The three pillars of this program promote making the Bible, nutrition, and exercise priorities in your life. Paying the right attention to these pillars will help sustain you in mind, body, and soul. Another way to ease your burden is to realize this is not a solo act, as one person cannot carry another through a difficult season. It takes a village of doctors, pastors, friends, and family to lovingly assist with recovery. As a caregiver, you will be much more effective as part of a team that takes shifts so that all may serve more effectively. This also helps you to have more energy to take care of yourself.

CHANGE YOUR LIFE

Week Six: Hope

We also glory in our sufferings, because we know that suffering produces perseverance; perseverance, character; and character, hope.

—*Romans 5:3–4 (NIV)*

For Your Soul

Do you believe the Lord has "plans to prosper you and not harm you, plans to give you hope and a future"?

Are you dealing with anxiety or depression? Are you getting the help you need?

First, as in all things, ask Jesus to heal you, and second, pray for wise counsel.

Have others storm heaven on your behalf!

Do you recognize that your symptoms are not your destiny? "The one who is in you is greater" than any of your symptoms.

Your problem is not permanent. No matter what age you are, your future has not even started.

Do you trust God enough to forgive Him, someone else, and (or) yourself?

Will you allow God to heal you? Will you allow Him to turn it to good?

How much of your future are you willing to waste on your past?

For Your Body

Listen to worship music to change your brain.

Meditate on God's Word in order to lift your mood and your life. Put key verses on your phone or on index cards. Start and end your day on a high note.

Listen or attend church services. You can always sit in the back.

Tune out excessive tech and media so you can tune into peace.

View food as a drug because it is. Eat the rainbow. Enjoy the healthy fats listed.

Get a physical and have your vitamin and hormone levels checked.

Move your body to uplift your spirit. Enjoy small, frequent doses of sunlight.

Focus on what brings you hope: your Bible, real food, and moderate exercise.

If you are grieving because of a current or past loss, you are not alone. Hope and healing are available through support groups nationwide.

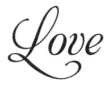

And now these three remain: faith, hope and love. But the greatest of these is love.

—*1 Corinthians 13:13 (NIV)*

Wе begin and end with love, because without love, the rest really doesn't matter. This final chapter focuses on love with regard to relationships and weight management, whether the relationship is with self, a significant other, a spouse, or a child.

You Will Never Be Perfect

Whoever does not love does not know God, because God is love.

—*1 John 4:8 (NIV)*

Unfortunately, many people seek out weight-loss programs because at some level they believe they are unlovable. Although our first love has not abandoned us, we don't always trust Him when it comes to finding and sustaining love. We believe we need to look a certain way in order to live happily ever after. Since most of us are not in the supermodel category, it is easy to blame our unlucky attempts at love on our physical appearance, ruining our self-esteem. In this search for love without God, many appear to be living a healthy lifestyle, but they are not. Both weight gain and weight loss can be a type of self-inflicted abusive behavior. There are countless women and young girls punishing themselves with eating disorders or over-exercising every single day.

Both single and divorced female clients have told me they believe their ideal mate could never love them just as they are. Perhaps a boyfriend or spouse left them for a younger, prettier, skinnier model, or they have abandonment issues from childhood. Whatever the case, these poor souls are striving for an unrealistic version of themselves. This distracts them from being who God created them to be. Since they are never satisfied, they continue to over-exercise and diet in search of the perfect body, which they believe will bring the perfect love.

If you have to go through unrealistic efforts for the supposed love of your life to be attracted to you, you will have to continue to jump through hurdles in order to keep it. This has zero to do with God's version of love. Besides wreaking havoc on your state of health, you most likely will get farther from your weight goal than closer because of unsustainable draconian efforts. You may think you are alone, with only a minority of women actually buying into this. However, if this were the case, we would not have multibillion-dollar industries profiting off of our insecurities. Although a healthy self-esteem involves wanting to look your best, without putting God first, even this can get distorted.

Plastic surgery is ubiquitous in Dallas. I have actually heard husbands tell their spouses, "Honey, if you want to get x done, Dallas is the place to do it." So many people get plastic surgery that when I was included in a picture with a group of three other women who were under forty at a former gym, I was the only one who had not had work done. On the other hand, like many, I have friends who have had plastic surgery as part of a healing process. I am not talking about healing. I am talking about going through this in order to get noticed. Sadly, these women do get noticed but often for the wrong reasons. Some women who have had the most work done seem to have the least amount of confidence because they are putting all of their confidence in their appearance. Without counseling, this only gets worse. It appears to my unscientific mind that men who are attracted to the "perfect" woman already have one foot out the door, since they are constantly in search of the next best thing. Hence, it is impossible to keep up. I have sat at the bedside of a woman who had multiple plastic surgeries for enhancements, and it was heartbreaking. Whether we are single or married, what message are we giving young boys and girls when we put all of our confidence in an appearance that never seems to measure up? A gym owner recently confided in me that there were girls in their teens at his gym that had already had work done because they competed in beauty contests. If we start with plastic surgery in our teens, where do we go from there? A healthy life does not come from starving, purging, plastic surgery, or over-exercising, which all result in less energy to serve the kingdom.

You Will Always Be Loved

If it is God's will for you to be married, then He already has your spouse picked out for you. He has to pick out the spouse, not you. If He has other plans for your life, no perfect weight or body part is going to change that. Either way, you are already loved. Our purpose is to love Him first, whether we are married or not. If marriage is His plan for your life, He may just be waiting on you. Everyone says they are looking for a mature and grounded person in their faith. The question is, Are you that person when it comes to your faith? I certainly was not for a long time. I can tell you firsthand you are not going to attract the type of person who is going to go to church with your family if you haven't graced the front walkway of your own church because your weekends are too busy lamenting not finding the right person. Are you looking for love in all of the wrong places? God may be waiting for you to love Him first. He was in my case. After prioritizing that relationship, you are then better off using your gifts, time, and energy to love your neighbor. You might just run into someone else who is doing the same. The spark should be the light of Christ that exists between two hearts. You can't beat those fireworks. All else is shifting sands.

GOD'S TIMING

I remember being over thirty and not married, which was considered old at the time! Most of my friends had walked down the aisle and were celebrating the birth of a baby or two. Even if I was not questioning what was wrong with me for still being single and over thirty, others were.

Meanwhile, a navy pilot friend of mine told me about the White House Military Social Aide program. I applied and was excited to interview. However, I did not get a call back. I was then transferred to Fort Detrick, Maryland, home of the Ebola virus. In addition to my fascinating work with wartime planning medical systems, I lived in Frederick, MD, which at the time was a 100 percent bedroom community. To put this in layman's terms, there were zero single people in Frederick (well, almost). On the plus side, I was surrounded by beautiful farmland. However, just like the cows, I felt a bit like I had been put out to pasture.

At this point, I prayed to the Lord and asked Him to either make me happy as a single person or send me someone "value added." I did not want another rescue mission. Does that sound harsh? My problem wasn't that I didn't want to help people. My problem was I did want to help people, and all of my energy had been poured into trying to fix a significant other, which meant not having a whole lot left over.

Can I get an Amen?

Of course, I needed some fixing myself since I was repeating unhealthy patterns from childhood. I was also a rescue mission. I am not implying that everyone that is single needs to be fixed. Jesus was single. I am just saying that I had some unresolved issues, which was hardly a surprise. In the meantime, we decided that there was a better way for me to spend my time than lamenting being single or continuing to make poor relationship choices.

Instead of face-planting into a tub of Ben and Jerry's every night, I began to read the Psalms every morning. Instead of going home to a lonely apartment after work, I decided to join the church choir. Instead of stuffing my face with popcorn, crying over late-night chick flicks on Friday nights, I went on long, beautiful bike rides on Saturday mornings, appreciating His creation. Instead of looking at families, lamenting whether or not I was ever going to have one, I taught Sunday school and served at local soup kitchens. This was also when I decided to go to counseling to deal with recurring negative childhood patterns that led to poor relationship choices. I decided to no longer allow my past to ruin my future. It was time to move forward from bad relationship groundhog day. I did the work, and so can you.

Then one day, out of the bucolic blue skies of Frederick, Maryland, the phone rang. Just as I was finally starting to embrace cow pastures, an unexpected curveball came my way. It was the White House calling to notify me that I had a second interview. It had been more than a year after my first interview. I thought that ship had sailed. Had they made a mistake? If I hadn't made the cut the first time, why was I going back for a second interview over a year later? When I finally decided to go in for this second interview, they told me I did very well on my first, but at the time, they had enough Navy personnel. Whatever the reason, it was not God's timing.

Many times in life we get a no and have no idea why, so of course we assume that it must be our fault. This often leads to unhealthy behaviors. We never think that just maybe it has something to do with God's timing. Almost two years to the date of my first interview and subsequent interviews/background investigation, I joined the program. It was so exciting to interact with the nation's best and brightest, one of them being my future husband.

I later realized had I gotten into the program when I first interviewed, I would have not met my husband, since he was stationed in Seattle at the time. These were typically two-year assignments due to military moves. The delay in timing allowed me to meet him. The delay in timing allowed me to mature spiritually and emotionally, leading to a healthier lifestyle. The delay in timing allowed me to go to counseling and heal from past hurts. The delay in timing was not a delay at all. It was God's timing. Could God have also been waiting on me? I only know that I needed to love God first before I was able to find the love of my life.

Not everyone is called to be married. Whatever your situation, seek the Lord first, then love your neighbor. In other words, "bloom where you are planted." Take the time to flourish while healing from past hurts, if needed. Being single is the least complicated stage of life, so take advantage of counseling if you need it! Then, if marriage does wind up being your calling, you have a better chance of being happily married for twenty years instead of being miserable for thirty or winding up in divorce court. Trust God's timing. His timing is better!

Love and Marriage

If I speak in the tongues of men or of angels, but do not have love, I am only a resounding gong or a clanging cymbal.

—1 Corinthians 13:1 (NIV)

Different stages of marriage have different challenges regarding weight management. What I am about to describe only applies to relationships that are not physically, emotionally, or verbally abusive. Those are in need of outside help, but they are still not beyond God's dominion. If you feel stuck in an unhealthy marriage, talk to a professional. The Bible's description of love has nothing to do with control, manipulation, or any other type of abuse.

Here are the three stages of marriage that I have noticed when it comes to weight management: endearing, smearing, and cheering. What stage are you in?

The first two stages of endearing and smearing are absolutes. You are either absolutely in love (endearing stage) with someone or they absolutely drive you crazy (smearing stage). Let's start with everyone's favorite: endearing. This is the stage of romantic love. You meet someone and wonder where this person has been all of your life. You forget to eat, or maybe you are too nervous to eat. You are majorly concerned about looking your best. This must be your soul mate! A few years and kids later, it is all you can do to squeeze into your sweatpants in order to drive to your local coffee shop after sleeping in on a Saturday morning, because you were up all night with a sick kid. Work, stress, family obligations, and other commitments have worn you down. Not only is it harder to maintain your weight, it is harder to maintain your marriage. Some marriages pull through this season triumphantly, while others do not.

The marriages that do not get stronger typically enter the smearing stage. Everything about the person that used to be charming is now unbearable. How could you have married someone that is your complete opposite? Let the smearing campaign commence! The smearing campaign may just be in your head, but many people are quite vocal about it. If you need more proof that you have picked the wrong person, just go to the authoritative source on all relationships: Facebook! See how much fun everyone else is having. Did she just post that her husband took her on a sunset cruise after watching the kids all day while cleaning the house and sending her off to the spa? You are convinced that there is something better out there, and everywhere you turn is a reminder. We can blame this on social media, but there is nothing new under the sun.

Too many people jump ship thinking that happiness is just around the bend with a different partner. If you jump ship because you are bored in your marriage, or are not in love anymore, you will wind up in the same boat with a different crew the next time around, surrounded by the survivors of the last shipwreck. Ask God to teach you how to love in the present, instead of pinning all of your happiness on an unknown future. Whoever your spouse is, he was not created to fulfill your every need in your current or future life. Only God can do that.

However, God can breathe new life into your marriage! You don't have to be on the brink of an affair. You just have to want to put Him at the center of your union. Just be ready to brace yourself for whatever happens next. You may not see change overnight, but eventually something will happen. You may also need to make some changes. Your efforts need to begin by praying with all your heart, mind, and soul for the Lord to walk alongside you and your spouse. Do not look for instant gratification. Do not expect every kind gesture that you go out of your way to do to be met with applause. That is not love either.

It is hard to invest in a relationship when you feel like you are the only one doing the investing. However, there is always room for improvement. You can start by cutting out sarcasm since this grows like a cancer. You might also plan a special event for your partner (like buying him tickets to a game, etc.) even though you feel like he or she is the one who should be initiating the change. You may invite another couple out for a double date, making it a fun night out, minus the pressure. When it comes to your marriage, you have to give it your best shot. My friend and counselor says even worse than being unhappy in a marriage is the regret many are left with in dealing with the aftermath, only to realize the grass was not greener. According to her, if you think counseling people through divorce is hard, counseling people through regret is worse.

The smearing stage isn't good for anybody. There are no winners either way. This is where people are either going to the gym to get super fit to the point of obsession or are drowning in food or alcohol to numb the pain. I can't tell you the number of clients who have come to me after gaining weight during or after a divorce. Many are either in divorce court or stuck somewhere in this seemingly never-ending process. If you don't know Jesus already, you can bet that you will be mentioning some deity once the legal bills arrive. Instead, your marriage may be able to survive and thrive, but first you need to humbly ask for help and accept answers you may not like.

The good news is that those who survive or bypass the smearing stage can eventually move on to the cheering stage! Yay! In the cheering stage, you celebrate instead of berate each other's differences. In the beginning, you may be the only one cheering, but positive reinforcement is good for everyone. This is not an absolute phase. You no longer think your spouse is an angel or the devil depending upon what mood you are in that particular day. You love the person for who they are, not who you want them to be. Marriage teaches us how to love in a self-centered world so He can increase while our egos decrease. The cheering stage is a joyful and peaceful stage.

More Peace Equals Fewer Pounds

You are not doomed to gain weight if you are unhappy in your marriage, but you are more likely to engage in unhealthy behaviors if you feel trapped. Whether you are single, married, or divorced, your confidence needs to come from the Lord, not another person. The more at peace you are with this concept, the more at peace you will be period. More peace equals fewer pounds. You are not a victim. You are a victor in Christ.

Instead of praying to be a size 0 in order to be loved, pray for peace. Jesus talked a lot about peace and forgiveness. Forgiveness also applies to marriage. You are not only called by your Father to ask for forgiveness, but you are also called to forgive your spouse and yourself. Seeking God first leads to a peaceful and happy marriage. Happy marriages are associated with longevity.

Weight Management and Your Spouse

If you have told your spouse to eat healthy and exercise and had a positive response, you are in the minority. In most cases, this does not go over very well. Occasionally there is a spouse who is health conscious and will respond favorably to a gentle reminder, but this is not the norm. Remember, "preach the Gospel at all times; if necessary, use words." You need to be your own best advertisement if you want to inspire others to get healthy.

When you see the Gospel in action, you cannot help but be attracted to it. When healthy living is pursued for the right reasons, it can have a similar effect. Studies show that when one spouse gets healthy, the other has a much higher chance to follow suit. So how do you get your spouse to eat healthy, careful to not suggest anything that might make him or her feel unattractive or unloved? A more successful approach would be to make comments about how much better you feel. Just smiling more makes a difference. Express love for your spouse through your newfound energy by offering to go for a walk or participating in a hobby he or she enjoys. Help out with one of his chores. People notice when someone has more energy, especially when they are willing to share it. It makes others want more energy, unless they have already given up. If this is the case, they need prayer.

> *If I speak in the tongues of men or of angels, but do not have love, I am only a resounding gong or a clanging cymbal.*
>
> —*1 Corinthians 13:1 (NIV)*

Nagging someone into making healthy choices backfires. Making ultimatums is even worse. It may take years for your spouse to want to make healthy choices, or it may never happen. Either way, your spouse is not an excuse for you not to take care of yourself. Your spouse's struggle actually requires you to pray for him or her as if you believe healing is possible, because it is. If you don't pray for him, who will? I have met many people that have written off their spouse and other family members from ever pursing a healthy lifestyle. Remember, someone could have just as easily written you off. Maybe they did. If it wasn't over this, it may have been over something else, so make the better choice and pray as if God is able to make this happen, because He is. It is not a prayer if you don't believe it can happen. Just like we don't want to be known for our lack of faith when it comes to ourselves, we don't want that to be our claim to fame when it comes to others. I have helped many men lose weight that I have never met after only working with their wives. Obviously somebody was praying.

Loving Our Children and Grandchildren

> *Can a mother forget the baby at her breast and have no compassion on the child she has borne? Though she may forget, I will not forget you!*
>
> —*Isaiah 49:15 (NIV)*

The only topic more emotionally charged than our own weight struggles is that of our children, which leaves many parents feeling guilty. In order to help your children, you have to first recognize guilt for what it is. Guilt is a tool of the devil. It renders you ineffective while breaking you down. Guilt does not help you or your children. It just wastes more time. Instead, when something touches a nerve, ask the Holy Spirit to empower you and your family to overcome it. Then believe it is possible in the name of Jesus. Don't forget to ask others to pray on your children's behalf. It takes a village of prayer warriors.

When it comes to our children's health, we can no longer wing it. The food and drink options in front of our kids today are bad, only to be coupled with sedentary entertainment. The only way around this is planning ahead. Exercise and healthy eating have to be a priority on a daily basis. This does not mean every meal has to be perfect or that your kids need to be exercising all day, but they need real food for most of their meals and snacks, and they need to keep moving. This may mean you driving to sports activities or carpooling. The good news is you do not have to sit while your kids are getting a workout. I have driven to hundreds of soccer practices over the years and worked out by either jogging or walking around the same field. At swim practice for my children, I used to swim in open pool lanes or use the gym that was available.

Working Parents

When it comes to healthy eating, few working moms have time to spend in the kitchen, but we still need to make sure our children are not eating junk all day. I do include practical ideas even if you eat out often. However, someone needs to manage what your children are eating and whether or not they are getting enough exercise. It most likely is not going to be them, as least not in the earlier years.

Although it is easy to get lured into distractions, you don't want to live with regret. Many people believe a career or some other carrot is holding the key to their happiness, leaving children to subsist on junk food and little exercise, only to find out that it was not worth it. Other full-time working parents have no choice and are already stretched thin. However, this chapter can help you make better choices within the same amount of time you currently have. There is no question raising children takes more time and effort than most of us could have ever imagined. However, if you don't get involved and put the time in up front, investing in your child's healthy eating, exercise, and activities, you may be forced to put the time in later, trying to put the pieces back together. This can show up as a weight problem, among other things. Start today; it is never too late!

Remember that God loves your children more than you do. Ask the Lord to help you make optimal choices for your children's spiritual, emotional, and physical well-being. Pay attention today so you won't live with regret tomorrow. Regret is unhealthy for all parties.

CHILDREN AND OBESITY

Make sure you check with your pediatrician before implementing any diet or exercise program for your child. There are licensed psychologists who specialize in children with eating disorders that can also help if needed.

I have zero credentials when it comes to working with children. Yet, because I am a certified personal trainer, I was occasionally assigned young girls as clients at the YMCA. These girls were between nine and eleven years of age. Since then, I have also worked with moms and their teenage daughters. The difference between the young girls I worked with at the YMCA and the moms and teenage girls I work with today is that the YMCA girls were under doctor's orders. Their parents were told that their daughters had to begin a supervised exercise program to lose weight as soon as possible. Although one of them weighed as much as I did at the start, the good news is that these girls were able to reach their goals.

With these girls, the first thing I did was find out their interests. Again, we are back to *why* they would want to pick up a carrot over a cupcake in the first place. Whenever working with anyone, whether it is a child or adult who is struggling, it is always helpful to find out someone's passions. By focusing on something positive while we exercised, it brought a positive association to our appointments. It also let them know I cared. This helped make the time spent with each child something they anticipated.

I am not a person who would gravitate toward a job working with children. You don't need to be a childhood expert either. I finally realized the main reason these girls enjoyed our time together was the attention and activity. It didn't matter what the activity was. We may have jumped rope and then done modified push-ups, Hula-Hooped, or did jumping jacks. Although not all children gravitate toward sports, almost all like activity. Children are more in tune with this than adults.

If I worked with a child who also liked sports, I would emphasize how healthy eating and exercise would help them perform better. I always tried to tie their interests to healthy eating and exercise, and taught how these changes would contribute to making them even better at whatever it was they enjoyed doing. Just like adults, kids also have a why. Children need to exercise every single day for a minimum of one hour. They also need to move throughout the rest of the day. We cannot depend on this to happen at school. With the girls I worked with, I strongly encouraged organized activities such as dance to keep them active if they were not into sports.

I actually believe most kids would eat healthy and move more if the options were more readily available than junk food and media. Instead, just like adults, when you have white flour and sugar around with more sedentary options than active ones, children are going to lean toward those. The reason children don't naturally gravitate toward healthy choices is because they have already eaten so much fast food that regular healthy meals don't seem to taste as good as fries and a shake. Since almost 50 percent of our meals as Americans are eaten out, even our kids have hyperstimulated palates. On top of that, most parents are not eating healthy at home. Throw media in the mix, and we have the perfect storm.

Although I would reinforce all of the information I shared with the girls with their parents, challenges became evident. I realized I was not taking on a child as a new client but rather an entire family. If one child in the house is eating differently from everyone else, there can be problems. This was another reason I felt led to create FAITH VS. WEIGHT for women. I purposely did not want to target children, although this is the area that grieves my heart the most. I target moms. This is not meant to be a guilt trip. This is meant to reclaim mom's health, which will benefit the entire family. As far as children are concerned, mom is where love originates. We all know that when momma is happy, everyone is happy! If I can get mom and eventually dad on board, kids will follow. It is much more difficult and unrealistic to target children when their choices are rarely within their control. As I used to say to the parents of my younger clients, "Your nine-year-old doesn't have a set of car keys." They eat what you bring in the house.

When working with children, focus on energy rather than appearance. Do not discuss scales or weight. Often, kids will voluntarily share their weight loss because of their excitement. Give kids hints on how to avoid feeling sluggish by eating their protein or veggies first rather than carbohydrates, which may cause them to overeat and feel tired.

WHAT TO EAT?

The same plan I recommend for adults, I recommend for children, with the following changes: Children can have one starchy carb at each meal. Remember, the recommendations for starchy carbohydrates are on the lunch/dinner chart. These are whole food options. Starchy carbohydrate intake is based on activity and growth, so children need the carbohydrates. If they are active, they can also have one starchy carb with their afternoon snack. Teenagers who are not overweight and very physically active will need more. How much? My uniquely finely tuned calibrated complex formula is this: is the child growing up or out? Out means it's time to cut down on the carbs, including sugar.

MEALS

In order to teach school-age children what their portions and proportions should look like, you can draw a plate and cut it in thirds. The first third is protein, the second is a vegetable or fruit, and the third is a starchy carb. Then choose foods for each of the thirds for breakfast, lunch, and dinner. Also choose a healthy fat. Tell them they can add a small amount of a plant-based fat as a topping or an add-on. It is easier to tell them to add it at the end, giving them a list of what one hundred calories of fat looks like rather than trying to show this on a plate. Fat comes in different sizes. In terms of volume, a hundred calories of olive oil looks very different from a hundred calories of guacamole. Plant-based fats are: one tablespoon of olive oil, two tablespoons of nuts, one tablespoon of nut butter, or one-fourth cup guacamole or hummus. I recommend smaller amounts for children under ten.

An exception to the one tablespoon of fat rule applies when eating peanut butter or nut butter sandwiches. In this case, two tablespoons of nut butter (even though one is recommended on this plan for adults) is recommended for children if that is their only protein. Two tablespoons of nut butter has enough protein to count as a protein for kids. A great addition is one half of a banana sliced, but a light smear of low-sugar jelly (approximately seven grams per serving) is fine. Carrots, celery, and cherry tomatoes on the side round out the meal. For additional protein, add one light string cheese as an option. In order to keep carbohydrates to one serving, go for thin sliced breads.

Bread Options

Bread options (all found in the freezer section) include: Alvarado ST. Bakery sourdough bread, or Food for Life Ezekiel 4:9 bread, low glycemic. Both are delicious sprouted grain choices. Alvarado ST. Bakery also makes a sprouted, diabetic lifestyles low glycemic bread. For a delicious gluten-free option, try gluten-free Canyon Bake House bread. If you are looking for two slices instead of one: Alvarado ST. Bakery sprouted flax seed bread and Dave's Killer Bread thin sliced with twenty-one grains are both low-calorie options, with two slices counting as one carbohydrate serving on this plan.

Breakfast

After hydrating with water, children of all ages and stages need breakfast. The hardest thing most parents struggle with is what to serve as a protein.

One option is to try the five-minute smoothies from the breakfast/snack chart, which seem to be a hit with both children and adults. Hard-boiled eggs are also easy, but not all children like them. Mine are picky when it comes to how their eggs are prepared. I finally realized they loved French toast, so I beat one egg per slice of one of the whole grain breads listed above and add vanilla extract. After thoroughly soaking the bread, I cook it on medium-high heat for five minutes in a small pat of grass-fed butter. I serve this with cinnamon and berries. If they want syrup, I drizzle one teaspoon. This is a great way to get your kids to eat whole grains and eggs. Although I would try to minimize processed foods as much as possible, nitrate-free turkey sausage is also an option. If your kids are not hungry for breakfast, make sure they are not eating late at night. If they are still not hungry, try different options. Mine are not hungry for scrambled eggs and oatmeal but love the French toast I just described.

SNACKS

The purpose of snacks for both children and adults it to keep fueled until the next meal. Test to see which snacks work best for your kids. The amount depends a lot on their rate of growth and activity level. Neither adults nor children want to approach dinner starving, because it will result in over-eating. The biggest problem, whether children are over or underweight, is grazing. The more substantial their snack, the less chance they will graze. This may mean a full sandwich after school, using two slices of regular sliced whole grain bread instead of thin sliced if you have growing teenagers, or a string cheese and an apple if you have preteens. If they don't want a sandwich but are still hungry, you can add a hundred calories (two tablespoons of nuts) to a string cheese and an apple. Snack suggestions for children that are less active or want a lighter snack are on the breakfast/snack chart.

DAIRY

Keep dairy to three servings a day. If they drink milk as one of their dairy servings, I recommend it at their evening meal since there is no reason to raise blood sugar early in the day. Grass-fed omega-3 dairy is your best option. Grass-fed yogurt is a good choice if it is plain without added sugar. You can then add berries and some nuts. A great way to naturally sweeten yogurt for kids (and adults) is to defrost frozen berries or warm them up in a microwave before putting them in plain yogurt. The juice from defrosted frozen berries acts like a sweetener. You can also add frozen berries to yogurt before they go to school, and they will be defrosted by snack time. Smoothies, as described in the breakfast/snack chart, work as an afternoon snack or breakfast.

DESSERT

Dessert is served after dinner. That is why it is called dessert! If a reasonable amount is chosen, kids can have what they want. I tell my children they can have whatever they want as long as they eat a reasonable portion size. Have them decide on the amount before they begin eating so they will learn what a reasonable portion looks like. Have them put it on a separate plate. Expecting children to stop eating a dessert that is not pre-portioned on a separate plate is as unrealistic as expecting adults to do it. Teach kids to have dessert after a balanced dinner instead of at random times during the day, as it makes a big difference in controlling sugar cravings.

Occasionally when we are out to lunch, my kids want ice cream when it is available. The key is to have them eat it after their meal. Sugar before a meal is never a good idea. I always ask them if they would rather have their dessert after lunch or after dinner. If they decide they really want it after lunch, they are not offered any after dinner. My goal is to teach them that one serving of sugar per day is more than enough. Controlling kids' sugar cravings also means weaning them off soda and juices. Replace these with unsweetened tea or water. Ginger-peach and pomegranate-flavored teas are appealing. There are many unsweetened options in the tea section.

Restaurants

Once children get the hang of this at home, have them draw a plate cut in thirds, and now talk with them about making choices at their favorite restaurants. Tell them that the amount of food at restaurants is going to slow them down and that they need to decide on their own amounts. Teach them to ask for a separate plate to create their own thirds from their bigger entrée, with some healthy fat added. If they are at a burger joint, they can get a single cheeseburger with a whole grain bun (if available) or small fries but not both. They can add lettuce, onions, pickles, and tomatoes. If they select small fries, tell them to skip the bun. They do not need to add an additional fat since fries are already cooked in fat. Watch the portion size on fries. A small fry today is the equivalent of what a large used to be only a few years ago. I always dump the extra fries.

Birthday Parties

There are certainly times to be more lenient, but that doesn't mean overdoing it. When my children were younger and went to lots of birthday parties, I emphasized one less slice of pizza if they were also going to have cake. However, I did not do this at the party, since this would have backfired. We discussed this before the party. It is not worth losing the war over one battle. I would ask them if they wanted cake at the upcoming party, and they would of course say yes. Then I would ask them how much pizza they thought they should have if they were also having cake. They usually would downsize the amount on their own. The point here is to get them to think, because whether it is a child or adult, when someone feels they have control over the decision, there will be greater compliance.

The Icing on the Cake

For young children's birthdays and celebrations, most people no longer have the time or expertise to bake a superhero cake. Why bother when you can buy a gorgeous cake with your kid's favorite character on it? The problem is the frosting. Most of these still contain unhealthy fats along with corn syrup and loads of sugar.

I am not suggesting that your child never eat birthday cake again, but what I am suggesting is for your house to limit the cake and cupcakes with frosting. Keep frosting to special occasions. A cupcake is not a health food just because it came from a health food store. Frosting is still loaded with sugar and fat. It used to be a special occasion when someone in the family baked a homemade cake made with real ingredients. Now, we eat vastly unhealthier versions as an all-day, everyday affair and don't even need an occasion. A fun way for toddlers to pace themselves is to have a contest to see who can make a dessert last the longest.

Middle School

Middle-school-age nutrition requirements are all over the map depending on a child's growth and activity levels. If kids are eating appropriate amounts of protein, veggies, fruit, and plant-based fats, they will usually self-regulate. Carbohydrate intake is tricky. Some need more to grow, and some will store it as fat if they are not as active. Since quality counts, whole grains are always a better option. Children going through growth spurts may need more than one starchy carbohydrate serving and protein at each meal, or they may need to turn their snacks into more of a meal. Eating reasonably portion-controlled meals more frequently is always better than overdoing it at one sitting.

Whatever the case, each snack and meal should include a high-quality protein and a vegetable or fruit. Healthy fats are not at the top of middle school kids' minds, but these are easy to include in the form of nuts at snack time or avocados, guacamole, hummus, or olive oil at mealtime. If these are served in appropriate serving sizes, according to age and stage, cutting down on carbs or increasing them will then depend on whether the child is growing up or out. Ensuring enough energy for play and growth without overdoing it is the goal.

Most days, I have my middle-school-aged boys pack their snacks and lunch for school. I want them to be in the habit of preparing and making healthy choices, which requires thinking ahead. No one else is going to do this for them, so they might as well start learning how to do it now. If you are overwhelmed by the idea of just trying to get your children out the door, no problem; just look at this as a summer project. It is a lot easier to implement things in the summer when you have more control of their schedule. The school year can be stressful enough.

TEENAGERS

With teenagers, it is even more important to find out their why—or they are just flat-out not going to do it. Drama, sports, or other interests can inspire them to kick it up a notch. Coaches may reinforce the fact that athletes are naturally faster when they are leaner. Lead roles in drama are easier to come by when you look the part. As bad as that sounds, I have heard this from many mothers of children in drama. The key here is to teach young men and women how to make healthy changes before they try draconian ones. However, if none of these things interest your teenager, something else will, or maybe already has.

Look for ways to emphasize how healthy eating and exercise can help them reach their goals. You can also have someone else teach these principles. Then you can reinforce the suggestions at home. Even if you are delivering the same message, they may need to hear it from someone else. Whether or not you are able to convert your teenager into choosing a healthy lifestyle, do not despair. You are still imprinting your healthy choices on their brain. They are watching you, and you are setting an example. I still remember how and what my parents ate, and I am sure you do too (whether it was good or bad). They may not fall in love with steamed spinach, but someday they might remember that you did.

Teenagers and Depression

I remember stopping at a roadside IHOP in Oklahoma one day with my family and being the only one who ordered an egg white omelet with veggies (light oil), and avocado on the side. As we were walking out, I saw a high school boy who was morbidly obese with a baseball cap pulled over his eyes. He was just hanging out in front of IHOP in no apparent rush to go anywhere, looking as if he had already given up on that particular day. Since then, I have seen many obese and morbidly obese children and young adults in Texas and Oklahoma. I realize other states have it even worse. Life is difficult enough without adding problems that are entirely preventable. These teenagers can lose the weight. Many do not know how or care enough to try because they do not have a reason that is big enough. They have already given up.

Depression is a significant factor for many overweight teens. However, trying to tackle an obesity problem without first addressing depression is more time wasted. Excessive media, drugs, alcohol, porn, and sexual promiscuity among teenagers make things worse, yet these are all more accessible when teens are not engaged in meaningful endeavors. Self-esteem-building activities, parental involvement, and counseling can help turn this ship around. However, it may take the kind of prayer that will not let go until there is a blessing. Even if your teen cannot be dragged to church, make sure you are going. Don't give up. You never know who or what might trigger your child to pursue a healthier lifestyle. It might even be you. Remember to ask others to storm heaven on your child's behalf.

For this reason, since the day we heard about you, we have not stopped praying for you. We continually ask God to fill you with the knowledge of his will through all the wisdom and understanding that the Spirit gives.

—Colossians 1:9 (NIV)

Be Realistic

With my children, I try to influence a minimum of two meals and one snack a day. It isn't always perfect, but I try to make sure that two out of three of the meals they eat per day are healthy, with at least one healthy snack. This way, if we wind up in a less than ideal situation for one meal, I don't stress out about it since the rest of the time they are fueling properly. Since there is no reason to overeat, I remind them to keep their portions in check.

If you have children who won't touch vegetables, put out raw veggies first with guacamole or hummus when they are hungry. Teach them what an appropriate amount looks like for their age, which is usually two tablespoons to a one-fourth cup, depending on their size. If you have to put cheese on veggies for them to eat veggies, put real cheese and be cognizant of the amount. Then put out protein and finally the starchy carbohydrate. Again, remember that carbohydrates are not bad. A person who sits at a desk all day but eats carbohydrates like he is training for an ironman is a different situation. Children should eat carbs based on growth and the energy they burn, and hopefully they are burning more than adults. It is just easier to regulate the amount if they have already had some protein first.

When I hear, "I'm hungry," and there is something tempting around, I always tell my children to eat a healthy meal or snack first, if they have not already, and to save the tempting item for dessert after dinner. If they recently ate or it is a time they are not normally hungry, then I know they are being tempted because it is there—just like adults. In both cases, it is best to save whatever it is for normal dessert time. It is much harder to control intake of sugar or white flour at random times a day or on an empty stomach, whether you are a child or an adult. Eating meals and snacks on a regular schedule makes a big difference. My kids forget to graze when I make a conscious effort to give them real food every few hours, which is exactly what I want to do. Grazing is not your friend. It typically means overdoing carbs or sugar, while falling short on protein, healthy fats, and vegetables.

There are certainly times I slack off with my kids. At brunch, which is usually only after a 5K or soccer tournament in my house, there is more leniency.

They can order their favorite item at our local breakfast hangout. However, I still tell them to eat an egg before they dig into their pancakes. Their muscles need protein for recovery, but this also helps them keep their blood sugar from going out of whack from the pancakes. If not eaten in the correct order, I might find them craving junk for the rest of the day.

When it comes to eating out, some parents have already sworn off all fast food. This is by far the better route. Unfortunately, I have not achieved this Master Jedi level. However, as in all things, my plate looks the same with regard to portions and proportions at any type of restaurant, whether it has a Michelin rating or it is a drive-through. I encourage my kids to do the same. We all need to learn to make the best of every situation.

Sugar Rivalry

Sometimes families have to deal with both under and overweight teenagers at the same time. This can be a sensitive issue. When I had an underweight teenager going through a growth spurt, I added additional carbs *and* increased the frequency of his meals. Three times a day, he ate two servings of carbs but always with a protein and veggie, or fruit, and a healthy fat. In the afternoon, I would make the same smoothie recipe provided on the breakfast/snack chart with an additional protein added in the form of another serving of greek yogurt or a raw pasteurized egg. One raw egg does not affect the taste. (See the end of this section for groups that should avoid eating raw eggs. My children were teenagers at the time they started having raw eggs in their smoothies.)

In the evening after a sports practice, I would add a nut butter and jelly sandwich on whole grain bread (regular instead of thin sliced bread, since the teen needed to gain weight) after dinner with a glass of milk. In order to make this happen, I did not always offer a starchy carbohydrate at dinner but would still offer a small dessert. This way the underweight teen was hungry enough to eat again after dinner, and everyone had the same amount for dessert. Underweight children and teens do not need more sugar. They need more real food, yet everyone enjoys dessert. Allowing the same small amount of dessert for under and overweight children also helps overweight children not feel as if they are being penalized because they are overweight.

With smoothies, you can add calories as described or not and tailor it to each teen's needs without it appearing as if anyone is missing out. The extra sandwich at night works for a teen who is legitimately hungry. It is not enticing enough for one who is not. Whereas, if you are offering the underweight teen ice cream at 9:00 p.m., suddenly everyone is hungry, including the teen who is overweight. There is no need to make this harder than it already is.

Even if a child or teen is underweight, I am anti-grazing. Grazing usually leads to more junk calories. Then, when it is time to have a meal, children and teenagers are not hungry enough for real food like protein and vegetables. Protein is important. In order to have an appetite, it is better to have a beginning and an end to meals and snacks, even when eating five times a day. I personally don't subscribe to underweight children and teens having milkshakes or extra junk food in order to gain weight. This doesn't send the right message to anyone in the family, yet many health care professionals have suggested this. In the short term, this may be the only alternative. However, whenever possible, it is always better to develop a child's palette to crave real food. The only way to do this is to serve real food, turning healthy snacks into healthy mini-meals when necessary. This way children and teens can eat the same food at the same times whether they are over or underweight, with adjustments to the amounts. An overweight teenager might stick to the smoothie on the breakfast/snack chart after school, whereas an underweight teen would have the same smoothie with additional protein added in the form of extra greek yogurt or the raw pasteurized egg mentioned above, *and* an extra sandwich after dinner. Using these strategies, we were able to have an underweight teenager gain ten pounds in six months while the normal-weight teen grew at a steady rate.

The only caution here is that if you do decide to use raw eggs in smoothies, there is a greater risk for bacterial contamination (Salmonella) than with cooked eggs. The only raw eggs I recommend are those that are pasteurized. However, even in this case, raw eggs still run the risk of being contaminated with bacteria. Besides those who are allergic to eggs, the following groups should also avoid raw eggs: infants, children, pregnant women, the elderly, and those who have compromised immune systems. Salmonella infection can lead to life threatening complications. Since anyone can be affected, seek your Physicians or Pediatricians advice on the matter. You can always add another protein, such as additional greek yogurt, cottage cheese, or nut butter. There are *always* options.

THE BIG PICTURE

Therefore I tell you, whatever you ask for in prayer, believe that you have received it, and it will be yours.

—*Mark 11:24 (NIV)*

Remember to thank God in advance. If weight is a struggle for your child, the most important ingredient is prayer. However, it is only a prayer if you believe God is able to do it. You have to believe in the possibilities for your children since they are unable to see them. Since you are competing against addictive tendencies, even with children, remember to play worship music in the morning. This sets the tone for the entire day.

Just like grown-ups, kids have to be inspired to want something bigger than a doughnut or the couch. When it comes to healthy eating, always put the veggies and healthy fat or protein out first when your children are hungry. Wait to put the rest of the food out. Otherwise your kids will always pick the macaroni and cheese, or chips and salsa, over the broccoli. Carbs are served last on this plan, even if the carbs are brown rice.

START SPORTS EARLY

Childhood participation in sports is on the decline in the US. Girls and children from lower-income families participate the least. The key is to start early. It is very intimidating to try out for a team when you are ten years old and everyone else has been playing the sport since they were four years old. Although many public schools have after-school sports programs, these usually don't kick in until middle or high school. For some kids, this is already too late. The YMCA is a great place to look for both sports and financial assistance for younger children.

Many parents have told me that their child does not like sports. I believe them. However, sometimes we have to give children a chance to like something before they have a chance to quit. If a child does not want to be active or participate in a sport, find another activity. If they do not want to be active at all, tell them they are welcome to sit and watch the activity with no media. Whenever someone in my house does not feel like doing something active, I give him the alternative of sitting it out with zero media. This usually inspires a change of heart. When it comes to something new, I usually have children try it at least three times. Even adults don't feel comfortable right off the bat. We all need more than one chance. Activities like dance and marching band count! Pray that your child gets more excited about a healthy activity and eventually less interested in junk food and junk media. Guide your child to try different sports. If you feel like you are late to the game, some sports are easier to jump in than others. A full summer of swim lessons or tennis lessons can help get kids up to speed. Cross-country running and track can also easily be tackled in the summer.

Although my middle-school-aged children already play sports, we all needed more indoor exercise during the hot summer months in Texas. So we recently signed up for a family membership at a boxing gym. The family that boxes together … well, you get the idea. Anything to keep moving!

ACTIVITY

Keeping kids busy is hard work, but it is a key to prevention on several fronts. Boredom and loneliness in children is the same as boredom and loneliness in adults, and many use it as an excuse to overeat or worse. I overate when I was in middle school to fill the gap, which in turn contributed to a lower self-esteem, which led to more bad choices. Instead, as children get proficient with their activities, they can build self-esteem while also making friends, which is a big deal at that age. My children might practice their instrument, get homework done, and attend a sports practice or exercise on our treadmill or bike at home (with prodding). As mentioned, children should be moving a minimum of sixty minutes per day. This makes them feel better about themselves. By the time they have finished homework, sports, music, and free time (which does include media), dessert almost becomes an afterthought rather than an all-evening affair. Full-time working parents can encourage their child to take up an instrument, choir, or sport. These practices are usually held after school, which makes it easier on working parents, while giving children something productive to do until dinnertime.

I tell my children that if they want to be faster, stronger, and have fewer problems later on, they need to make good choices today. My children have also seen what happens when adults do not make good choices, and this is probably a better teacher than anything that comes out of my mouth.

Love the Lord Your God

Our Lady of the Coffeehouse

A neighbor used to tell me jokingly that on Sundays her family would go to Our Lady of the Coffeehouse. She avoided church since she did not want to force religion down her children's throats, so the local coffeehouse became their Sunday hangout. If the topic of God ever came up, He was treated as part of a history lesson. Unfortunately, this is becoming more and more common. This lie from Satan, disguised as the good intention of *empowering* our youth for tomorrow, is leaving them without hope for today (or tomorrow). A child in a poor family who knows Jesus has more hope than a child from an affluent family who has everything going for them by this world's standards but does not believe at a fundamental level that there is a God they can trust. We struggle enough as adults. Where are these children supposed to go for comfort? Perhaps this is another factor behind the childhood obesity epidemic. Our children are anxious.

> *Jesus said, "Let the little children come to me, and do not hinder them, for the kingdom of heaven belongs to such as these."*
> —*Matthew 19:14 (NIV)*

Bibles and Breakfast

After being born again, I used to put out a glass of water and Bible for each one of my sons. I wanted them to be in the habit of drinking water and reading the Word of God when they first awakened. As I prepared breakfast, I asked them to read a Bible verse or passage. As we now sometimes have more intense schedules or different departure times, I ask them to read a verse in the car using their Bible apps on their phones, while I drive them to school. Sometimes I get one line, and sometimes I get an entire passage.

It doesn't matter. I am just happy that the Word of God is going into their brains and coming out of their mouths, while penetrating their hearts. This always leads to discussion. At night, I remind them to pray, starting with the Lord's Prayer. I want their day, in the morning and evening, to be bounded by the Word of God because this is what God wants.

> *These commandments that I give you today are to be on your hearts. Impress them on your children. Talk about them when you sit at home and when you walk along the road, when you lie down and when you get up.*
>
> *—Deuteronomy 6:6–7 (NIV)*

Redeemed

> *Who gave himself for us, that he might redeem us from all iniquity, and purify unto himself a peculiar people, zealous of good works.*
>
> *—Titus 2:14 (KJV)*

Because my mother had to work full-time while pursuing additional education in order to gain job stability, my brother and I were left with unlimited and unsupervised free time. This combination led to me getting involved with the wrong crowd. It had gotten to the point where I needed committed parental supervision, or I was going to be sent to a place for troubled youth. My father could not live with the thought of me being sent away, so he stepped up, and my brother and I went to live him. At first, I dreaded the idea of living with my father because of past memories, but something seemed different about him. He had started to go to church, and it was starting to change him.

However, by the time we went to live with him, my heart was already hardened. I was angry and depressed. Drugs had become a big part of this equation, along with their associated behaviors. It took a couple of years before I found direction and peace. Although I did not make it easy on anyone, including my brother, my father refused to give up on me. He taught me that parenting was not a part-time job and that he was in it for the long haul. He apologized for the past and still struggled in certain areas but was learning to lean more on God every day. Eventually I did too. This was the only way we got through it. This never would have happened had he not stepped foot in a church. This was the first step for all of us. We would not have had a chance without it. My father taught me love through perseverance.

Jesus changes lives, even those of spouse abusers, unreachable teenagers, and those dealing with addictive behaviors. In this case, he did all three. I witnessed my father change, and eventually I did to. If you are struggling with your past or with teenagers, regular church attendance is nonnegotiable. Church cannot be an occasional stop when you have the time. I was dragged to church every week, and I now thank God for it. However, had I not seen what was talked about in church being lived out, it would have made matters worse. Ask God to help you be the person and parent you need to be. Finally, keep your eyes fixed on Jesus and do not give up. He never has, and He never will. Never underestimate the life-changing power of His love.

Many years later, my family and I were born again in the Lord Jesus Christ. This has been the only complete and transformative healing I have ever known. The Lord has given me a new heart, and it is joyfully and wholly devoted to Him.

Therefore we have been buried with him by baptism into death, so that, just as Christ was raised from the dead by the glory of the Father, so we too might walk in newness of life.

—Romans 6:4 (NRSV)

Change Your Brain

Bad News and Our Kids

All your children will be taught by the LORD, and great will be their peace.

—Isaiah 54:13 (NIV)

What are your children listening to when they are not in school or at church? Many households have the news on all day, every day, not realizing every word is subconsciously being soaked up by their children. Children do not have the emotional intelligence to deal with this amount of bad news or its severity. If you think our kids are not negatively affected by the constant media dump of bad news, you are wrong.

Children with ADHD are permitted to use a fidget spinner to manage stress, anxiety, fidgeting, and so on in the classroom, but everyone else uses them too. Spinners calm people of all ages down while helping them to focus. I'm all for that, but it grieves me that we have so many ten-year-olds that are already stressed out. We need to talk to children about healthy boundaries and safety, but we also need to allow them to be children. No one needs to listen to bad news all day, every day, especially not our children. Limit the types and amount of news on in your home so your children won't be tempted to use food as a comfort source.

Tech and Kids

All things were made through him, and without Him nothing was made that was made.

—John 1:3 (NKJV)

Although the Bible is an old book, it still is the authoritative source on parenting, even when it comes to technology. Don't kid yourself into thinking that the problems our kids face today have made the Bible irrelevant. The problems we face today as parents are still the same old problems. They are, as one of my children's teachers used to say, "like putting lipstick on a pig." Media may make evil more accessible and encourage inactivity, but at the end of the day, it is still a choice. If children do not know God, they won't know how to listen to Him and will be listening to everything and everybody else.

> *Behold, I send you out as sheep in the midst of wolves. Therefore be wise as serpents and harmless as doves.*
>
> *—Matthew 10:16 (NKJV)*

A Bucket of Books

When my children were younger, I decided not to have media in the car. Entertainment for my children was a bucket of books from the library, along with their children's Bibles. I paid many a late fee at the library and dealt with the shame of having to replace a few library books, but it was worth it. Library time was the only time I told my kids to get whatever they wanted, as long as it fit in the bucket. Now in their middle and high school years, my boys are as much, if not more, into tech as the next kid. However, I held out as long as I could, and it made a difference. There are still times when we are driving and I tell them to just read a book, because it's time to take a break from gaming. With books now on their phones, we no longer have a bucket of books, but they are always calmer after reading than when they are gaming. If you are a new mom, try to at least keep your car a media-free zone for as long as you can. There is zero incentive for children to read when they can passively be entertained instead. If you have young children, consider getting a container for your car. Then have your children pick out books from the library to fill that container. In a vehicle, you have a captive audience. I wonder how many children would have better attention spans and test scores if they had nothing to do but read.

Eat for Energy

The best example you can give others, including your kids, is to eat healthy yourself. Like it or not, we are live reality television. Our children watch our every move. My kids see me eat the same at home as I do at restaurants, with few exceptions. They also know that I will not go to a restaurant that does not serve vegetables or has only fried options. My philosophy with sugar in my house is out of sight equals out of mind. This applies to all age groups. Each person picks one or two favorites, which are placed in a drawer until it is time to have dessert. It doesn't need to be visible all day to tempt us because this usually leads to more servings than initially intended. How can we expect our kids to show restraint when we are not able to exercise it ourselves?

Do You Eat Like a Child?

> When I was a child, I talked like a child, I thought like a child,
> I reasoned like a child. When I became a man, I put the ways of
> childhood behind me.
>
> —1 Corinthians 13:11 (NIV)

A lot of adults still eat as if they are children. I cannot eat like my boys who are in their early teen years. If a team has ice cream after a soccer tournament, I don't get ice cream because I didn't just burn through the hundreds of calories they did. If you really want ice cream, have it at home in a hundred-calorie portion after dinner. Do not fall into the human garbage disposal trap of eating whatever is left on your kids' plates or eating whatever they eat. I understand not wanting to waste food, but we are in more danger of wasting our health when we eat high-caloric kid fare. Upgrade your eating habits to your age and current activity level. This is not a curse but a blessing.

Make Your Move

Sleeping with the Enemy

I repeatedly hear how one spouse is more of a negative influence on children than the other. Obviously this is not the case in every household, but it does come up more often than not. A parent doesn't mean any harm when they come home with doughnuts. This is their way to show love. However, since we now have a childhood obesity epidemic, we have to find other ways to show love. My favorite is walking and talking. Walking the neighborhood while talking is free and easy. You can bring a furry friend along and hear things from your children you may not hear otherwise. Believe it or not, this works into the teen years. Other ways to have fun with movement as a family is signing up for a 5K. You do not need to run; many people walk 5Ks. You also have the option to start with a one-mile fun run. Family bike rides can be a lot of fun also. Taking younger kids to a park allows them to run around and play with other kids. At home, you can have a Hula-Hoop competition during commercial breaks to see who can keep it going for the longest. You can also have children come up with active games. Whenever you can, get moving outside. God has a beautiful world out there just waiting for you to enjoy! There is a proven increased sense of well-being when you are out in nature. This is no accident.

For you shall go out in joy, and be led out in peace; The mountains and the hills Shall break forth into singing before you, And all the trees of the field shall clap their hands.

—Isaiah 55:12 (NKJV)

Set a Family Goal

My husband and I had the opportunity to take our children on their first trip to the Washington, DC, area. Although we were only in town for a few days, on our way to a wedding at the Naval Academy, we wanted to give our boys an overview of the national monuments. We could have taken the metro, busses, taxis, or some other form of transportation. However, we really didn't want to stand in endless lines just waiting to get information or a seat. So we made it our goal to jog the major national monuments. It had been a year since I had recovered from my gallbladder surgery and broken leg, so I wasn't sure if I would be up to the task. In total, our family had sustained five broken bones and three surgeries in the five years leading up to that trip, so I wasn't sure if the rest of us would be up to the task either. However, we slowly started training for local 5Ks, and we were building endurance. This wouldn't have happened if we hadn't worked at it one meal, one workout, and one physical therapy appointment at a time. We had to get the horse ready for battle in order for the victory to be the Lord's.

Sharing the Washington, DC area with our children was like traveling back in time since that is where my husband and I met. To be able to run the same route many years later, and with our children, was an experience I cannot easily put into words, especially after our recent health challenges. Although my husband was still in top running form, I was not able to run the same times, but at least I was ambulatory! If you had seen us the year before in varying stages of recovery, you would have thought our family jogging the monuments was a longshot, and you would have been right. Yet there we were, living in victory! We took plenty of breaks and pictures, so it was not laborious. As a matter of fact, I would have to say it was glorious! I will never forget that day. It was one of the happiest of my life.

Whether you are interested in jogging the monuments or not, there may be another active trip you have always wanted to take with your children, but up until this point, you were not sure you could do it because of excess weight or inactivity. If we were able to do it after five broken bones and three surgeries in the years leading up to our trip, so can you! Give yourself a solid year and go for it! Even if a year passes and you are not all exactly where you want to be, you can still be significantly better off than you are today. You may even surpass your initial goals. As my first navy recruiter said to me when I was contemplating applying for a scholarship program, with my then less-than-stellar academic background, "Shoot for the moon. Even if you miss, you'll land among the stars."

Take a Stand

Let us not love with words or speech but with actions and in truth.

—1 John 3:18 (NIV)

My primary reason for writing this book is to empower you and your children (and grandchildren) to have more energy to put Christ's love into action. I do not want my family to miss out on opportunity to share the love of Jesus Christ because we are either in a food coma or spending all of our time at the doctor's office. This plan has helped families get more energy to share Christ's love. It can do the same for you and your family.

Beyond healthy eating and exercise, the Lord also gives you more energy when you use it to serve others. As you serve others, your family will be positively affected in two ways. First, it will make them want more energy because they will see how serving others has positively affected you. They will eventually catch on to the fact that in order to get more energy, they need to take care of their health and serve. Second, there will also be a transfer or energy. As you have more energy to serve your family, you make a positive impact on the world, transferring your energy through them. This is your greatest legacy.

Love Your Neighbor

Loving your neighbor as a family can be a lot of fun. For the past three years, Prestonwood Baptist Church (PBC) has been one of the hosts for the Tim Tebow, Night to Shine, Special Needs Prom, held in all fifty states and sixteen countries for people with special needs, aged fourteen and older. Check it out! This is a first-class prom with volunteers stationed along a red carpet where guests enter the event. There are lights and cameras, but the best part is the action. We shout the name of each special needs guest while clapping as if they are royalty, because on this night they are. The joy I see in the eyes of our guests when they get a reception that this world does not commonly afford them rivals anything I have seen on any White House receiving line. Beyond the obvious reasons to love this event, my favorite part is volunteering with both of my boys, acting like a fool, especially with my youngest son, and basically jumping up and down while cheering. Both the young and young at heart can really enjoy volunteering!

Our family had another opportunity to share the love of Christ by making a joyful noise as we went Christmas caroling at a local hospital. Last year, the same group, Chi Sigma, a parent/student service organization, participated in Christmas caroling at a local nursing home, among one of its many outreach programs. My boys enjoyed passing out Santa hats to the residents. Christmas caroling is guaranteed to bring smiles to all ages!

When you are a fool for the Lord, you will be far less worried about making a fool of yourself. If singing is not your thing or jumping up and down on the red carpet, the options to share the love of Christ as a family are endless: soup kitchens, tutoring younger children who are at risk, mission trips, church fundraisers, or sponsoring a child. Volunteering is linked to longevity.

CHANGE YOUR LIFE

Week Seven: Love

It always protects, always trusts, always hopes, always perseveres. Love never fails.

—1 Corinthians 13:7–8 (NIV)

For Your Soul

Single/Dating

Do you love God first?

Is there too much emphasis on how you look and not enough on spiritual growth?

Do you trust God's timing with your relationships?

Are you as strong in your faith as the person you want to marry?

Are you seeking out wise counsel to heal from past issues?

Are you looking for love in all of the wrong places? Pursue the Lord first. Then use your gifts to serve the body of Christ. The Holy Spirit may wind up putting the right one right next to you.

Are you living a healthy lifestyle? Like attracts like.

The Married Life

Are you in the endearing, smearing, or cheering phase of your marriage?

Ask God to be the center of your marriage if you haven't already.

Ask for the Lord to help your spouse with his/her weight issue if needed. Ask God to help your spouse love you through whatever your issues are.

Children

Teach your children about Jesus. They need His peace just as much as we do.

Dump the guilt. Seize your opportunities.

Is there something distracting you from ensuring that your children are eating healthy and exercising that you can live without? Regret is unhealthy, so avoid it.

If your children are struggling, ask God to help, believing that He can.

Show your children what a healthy plate looks like. Ask them what they would choose to put on their plate, empowering them to make healthy choices.

If they are not responsive to healthy eating and exercise suggestions from you, get outside help, especially if depression is a possible factor.

Make sure healthy eating and exercise are the most attractive options available. Otherwise they will pick the path of least resistance.

Teenagers

Ask God to help you set the right example. Drag your teenager to church if you must. Be consistent. Seek counseling if needed.

Whatever the age, help your children find self-esteem-building activities. "An idle mind is the devil's playground."

A word from the Bible with breakfast is a great start to a loving conversation. The Bible tells us that the Word of God will not go void.

Play worship music in the mornings, as this sets the tone for the day.

For Your Body

Set an example of reading the Bible, eating real food, and exercising consistently. Even if your children are no longer listening, they are still watching, and so is your spouse.

Enjoy family time: walking, biking, swimming, 5Ks, hiking, boxing, or hitting the parks.

Use your energy to be the hands and feet of Christ as you serve your family. That energy will be multiplied through them to serve the world. This is your greatest legacy.

Look for opportunities where you can volunteer as a family. You will always reap more than you sow.

Conclusion

The commandments of the LORD are right, bringing joy to the heart.
The commands of the LORD are clear, giving insight for living.

—*Psalm 19:8 (NLT)*

God's laws are not given to oppress our lives but to bring "joy to the heart"! The seven virtues discussed in this book help us to follow His laws with clear "insight for living." If you need to repeat a week, repeat a week. This is not a pass/fail. The "Change Your Life" section at the end of each chapter is meant to be a refresher course for as many times as you need it. Here are a few highlights to help you succeed on your path:

Prudence. Ask yourself, "What is the most likely outcome of what I am about to do," *before* you do it. Put the Lord first. Is what you are about to eat going to give you energy or rob it? Instead of feeling like you are being pulled like a tin can on the back of a just-married getaway convertible, plan ahead. More days than we like to admit, we do have control over our food choices.

Temperance. Are you focused on God's power or on your limitations? Inanimate objects have no control over you. If you are having a hard time being temperate with a particular choice, it may belong in the prudence category. What has food done for you lately? Sugar ages you in more ways than one. This is not the Last Supper, so keep desserts to one hundred calories. Eat real food.

Faith. Do your food and exercise choices reflect your faith? Would your faith in this area touch Jesus? Pay attention to how your faith affects your decisions. Why can't it be you? Who do you limit when you believe you cannot do something? Point to yourself first. Then point to God. Faith is contagious. "Fitness doesn't start in the gym." Remember to exercise for your body type.

Justice. Put your need for God above your need for justice. Take God at His Word. 1) Love yourself as much as you love your neighbor so you can love more neighbors. 2) Thou shalt not covet thy neighbor's skinny jeans. 3) Forgive as the Lord has forgiven you, whether you feel justice was served or not. Trust God. Stress-free does not equal fat-free. Balance your eating and exercise.

Perseverance. Expose your excuses when it comes to exercising. Perseverance is not a feeling. It is one of the rewards of the fruit of the Spirit. Work on observation instead of condemnation. Are you worshipping God in the high places, as described in Habakkuk, basking in His glory? Underline the word *power* every time you find it in the Psalms. The battle is the Lord's. So is the victory.

Hope. Do you believe God wants to give you a hope and a future? Talk to God about any lack of trust or anger. Your symptoms are not your destiny. Get help if you need it. How much of your future are you willing to waste on your past? Forgive God, others, and yourself. Tune into worship music. Tune out media. View food as a drug. Make it work to your advantage. Eat the rainbow and incorporate the fats listed. Unhealthy choices make you feel worse, leading to a downward spiral. You are never going to experience a sustained improvement in your mood without corresponding improvements in diet and exercise. If you are grieving, find a Christian support group. This does not drag the process out; it facilitates it.

Love. Is God your first love? Do you trust God's timing with relationships? Are you in relationship groundhog day? If so, get counseling. Is your marriage in the endearing, smearing, or cheering phase? Ask God to be the center of your marriage. Get help if you need it. Teach your children about Jesus. Find a way to incorporate Bible time into family time. "Preach the Gospel at all times. If necessary, use words." Actively serve as a family.

Ask God to help you be a good example when it comes to making healthy choices regarding your faith and your weight. Expose and encourage your children to experiment with different interests (including active ones) until something sticks. Don't allow junk food and media to steal their confidence or their childhood. If depression is an issue, seek counseling. Giving up is not an option. Pray as if your life depended on it. God hears. He loves your children even more than you do.

As I conclude this book, I pray you may hear the same words from Jesus that He spoke to the woman He healed in the crowd, except with your name inserted below:

"_____, YOUR FAITH HAS HEALED YOU."

FAITH VS WEIGHT

Afterword

The inspiration for FAITH VS. WEIGHT came when I was as a young navy officer stationed at the National Naval Medical Center in Bethesda, Maryland. The city and hospital were named after a local church that took its name from the same place in Jerusalem where the invalid was healed. I served as an aide to the admiral of this five-thousand-member bustling command and as a military White House social aide. I was surrounded by executive-level leadership along with many of our nation's best and brightest at various White House events. From a career standpoint, this was a once-in-a-lifetime opportunity.

While at Bethesda, I also had an opportunity to volunteer to serve Communion on the cancer ward. It was a sacred privilege to share in people's lives at their most vulnerable moment. There was no pretense. If there is a time you are looking for God, this is it. Since cancer doesn't discriminate, our patients were all ages. As I wondered, *What if we could turn back the clock and intervene before things got to this point?* my time volunteering on the cancer ward taught me two lessons.

LESSON ONE: SEIZE THE DAY

One afternoon, I ran into an old friend from my early enlisted days. He was the same age as I. We were now both lieutenants. I was so happy to see him yet crushed that it was under these circumstances, with him being a patient fighting for his life. Thankfully, he pulled through, got married, and went on to bike across the US. There is nothing like staring death in the face to get you to start living.

LESSON TWO: THIS IS THE ONLY DAY YOU HAVE

I often ran into a beautiful young mom who prayed almost daily in the chapel. In her case, her days were numbered. Not a moment to waste. Yet she had a peaceful countenance about her that comforted all she came in contact with. This begs the question: How do people feel after they have had an encounter with us? Are we going to leave the world a better place than how we found it? Our days are also numbered. Today is the only day we have to make a difference.

Although I thoroughly enjoyed my day job, I actually learned more about what really mattered in life on the cancer ward. Not all disease is nutrition and fitness related, but the odds favor a much higher quality of life for you if you take care of your body. Instead of blaming your circumstances, this newfound energy can actively be spent making a difference serving the body of Christ. Because of this, I asked the Lord to give me the opportunity to one day serve on the preventative end of health care, before it was too late. Ten years and a few moves later, that time finally came.

My family and I moved from the San Francisco Bay Area to Dallas Fort Worth. Not being a native Texan, three things kept haunting me:

The higher incidence of overweight and obese adults and children, along with the associated health risks at younger and younger ages. I knew this was the case intellectually, but seeing it was a different story. It grieved me, because I saw a certain lack of joy and felt people giving up before they had even gotten started.

The second thing I noticed was the amazing faith this part of the country weaves into its life on a daily basis. Having lived in various parts of the US and overseas as a navy officer, I had never experienced such a vibrant faith-based community. This was not my first time in the Bible Belt. However, this was the first time I noticed faith, beyond the walls of churches, impacting so many facets of life. There was no lack of faith. Because of this, I started wondering why a significant number of people with such tremendous faith were not applying their faith to their weight problem. The next thing I noticed gave me an idea as to why this was occurring.

The highways into Dallas seemed to have the same three billboards over and over again. Different companies but the same message: bariatric surgery, weight-loss programs, and plastic surgery (in case you want to remove the excess skin after your weight loss). Since then, I have even seen signs advertising bariatric surgery for sale. This was and is big business (no pun intended). Not exactly a view of the Golden Gate Bridge. It seemed as if weight was a problem that could only be fixed at a high cost with medically supervised intervention.

I thank God for the gifted medical professionals who in many cases have saved lives because of these programs and bariatric or related surgeries. However, it is tragic that so many people believe expensive medical treatments or surgery are the only way out of this mess. With all the research, think tanks, government task forces, and organizations trying to fight this battle, is this the best we've got? I recently read an article supporting bariatric surgery as a "cure" for diabetes. It has dramatically improved this situation for many, yet I couldn't help thinking we need to intervene before we get to this last resort. I make this point not to hammer bariatric surgery. It exists because there is a market for it—just like there is a market for diet pills, shots, and shakes.

It was at this point that I certified as a personal trainer specializing in women's health and weight loss. FAITH VS. WEIGHT was launched in Coppell, Texas, at the Coppell Family YMCA.

*Jesus came and told his disciples, "I have been given all authority
in heaven and on earth. Therefore, go and make disciples of all the
nations, baptizing them in the name of the Father and the Son and
the Holy Spirit. Teach these new disciples to obey all the commands I
have given you."*

—*Matthew 28:18–20 (NLT)*

It wasn't until I was born again and teaching FAITH VS. WEIGHT at
Prestonwood Baptist Church in Plano, Texas, that I realized there was an
even bigger issue at stake than just keeping people out of hospitals. As a
Christian, when you are immobilized because of health issues or your weight,
this affects at least two people. You and whoever you were going to share the
Gospel with that day but couldn't, either because of compromised health or
weight-related issues, or from just being too tired to get up off of the couch,
because you are in lousy shape.

You and I are not the only ones who need to be healed. The reason we need
energy to serve the kingdom is to fulfill God's call to spread the Gospel. In
the Bible, once people were healed, they could not keep their mouths shut
about Jesus. Neither should you! As you heal, you can help others heal as you
tell them about Jesus. You need energy to do this. One woman in the Bible
told an entire village about Jesus! She was not responsible for whether or not
they received Him, but they did.

*They said to the woman, "We no longer believe just because of what
you said; now we have heard for ourselves, and we know that this
man really is the Savior of the world."*

—*John 4:42 (NIV)*

The Mission Field

So as you reclaim your newfound energy, where do you start? Where is your
mission field? One night after leaving one of my son's soccer practices, I
got my answer. Somehow when we left, I took a wrong turn. As soon as I
realized I was heading in the opposite direction, I tried to make a U-turn.

However, with every chance I might have had, there was another no U-turn sign. Eventually I landed in a church parking lot finally headed in the right direction. Then I saw a sign that was only visible when leaving the church. It was pitch-black at night, but the sign's bold letters seemed to call out to me as they were vividly illuminated by my headlights: *You Are Now Entering the Mission Field.*

Whether we are aware of it or not, the mission field exists as soon as we walk outside our front door (in some cases, we don't even need to leave home). This is it. You and I are the light of the world. If we are unable to be the hands and feet of Jesus, showing His love through our actions, then who else is going to share the Gospel? You can make this world a better place by loving the Lord first, which teaches you how to love yourself so that you can have the energy to love others and share the good news with a world that desperately needs it, before it is too late.

When I first realized I was surrounded by the mission field, I felt overwhelmed, struck by my inadequacy to make any difference at all. Then I remembered I was not alone. First, the Lord provides wisdom through the Holy Spirit, who inspires us with the right word at the right time, if we ask for it. Second, the Lord provides through His church. The church is designed to equip us for the mission field: through the Word of God; through the Godly example of others already serving; and through the fellowship of other believers. You and I are not meant to go it alone, but we still have to go forth, right here, right now. This is why we need more energy.

I pray this book has helped you and will continue to help you magnify His glory by reclaiming your energy to serve the kingdom boldly, wherever your mission field happens to be.

"Behold, I am with you always, even to the end of the age."

—*Matthew 28: 20 (WEB)*

Prayer for Salvation

If you declare with your mouth "Jesus is Lord," and believe in your heart that God raised him from the dead, you will be saved.

—*Romans 10:9 (NIV)*

If you or someone you meet while serving in your mission field has not accepted the Lord Jesus Christ as a personal Savior, consider what is being abandoned for now and into eternity. You need a Savior in order to be saved.

In your own words, with all of your heart, you can embark on a personal relationship with the Lord Jesus Christ today. You can be saved. If you have already been born again, you can help someone else who has not received this same gift. Here is a place to start ...

"Jesus, I need You. I finally realize that living my life my way without You is not living life at all. I am a sinner, and I am sorry for my sins. I know You died on the cross to rescue me from these sins. This is a debt I can never repay. I know God raised You from the dead, so I could have new life, and I am ready for it. Lord of my life, I am excited to follow You with all of my heart. I want to be with You both now and in eternity. I know You are the only path to salvation."

For "Everyone who calls on the name of the LORD will be saved."

—Romans 10:13 (NIV)

Congratulations on taking your first step in pursuing the greatest love of your lifetime! Like any relationship, you will want to spend time growing in your commitment. First, start with praise, thanking the Lord Jesus Christ for all He has done for you. Then ask Him to help you and anyone else who needs prayer. He is interested in every facet of your life, so ask for help on this journey. Finally, pray for those who do not know Him.

Now it's time to find a church that actually teaches the Bible. Why go to church if you can hear the same thing from a motivational speaker at work? This is humankind's approach, not God's. Instead, seek out inspiration from God's Word. How can you tell if a church is teaching the Bible? Start reading your Bible. Some churches teach just the parts most people want to hear. However, we only grow when we hear the whole story. When I was born again at the age of forty-seven, I felt I had some catching up to do. I was not just hungry for God's Word. I was starving. Bible studies at church were the catalyst for me, both in accepting the Lord Jesus Christ as my personal Savior and in getting to know The Great I Am.

If it weren't for Chrissie Dunham, director of Women's Ministry at Prestonwood Baptist Church, inviting me to find out more about receiving Christ, and Suzy Bastian, teacher of the New Christians class, and the Amazing Collection, I would still be lost, driving around some church parking lot in circles. Tell someone.

APPENDIX

THE FAITH VS WEIGHT DIET

TIMING

Wake Up
Drink water with a half a lemon

Good Morning, Jesus
Coffee or tea with cinnamon

Breakfast
See Breakfast/Snack chart (protein/fat/fruit or vegetable)

Drink Water

Snacks (AM is Optional)

Drink Water

Lunch
See Lunch/Dinner chart (protein/fat/vegetable)

Drink Water

Snacks PM
See Breakfast/Snack chart (protein/fat/fruit or vegetable)

Drink Water

Dinner
See Lunch/Dinner chart (protein/fat/vegetable)
Enjoy water with lemon or lime

Less Active Option (Dinner Only)

To your protein, fat, and vegetable:
1.   Add one-hundred calories SC* plus one-hundred calories dessert
2.   Or add two-hundred calories SC* and skip dessert
3.   End with decaf coffee or herbal tea then stop eating

More Active Options (Dinner Plus After Dinner Snack)

To your protein, fat, and vegetable:
1.   Add one-hundred calories SC* and skip dessert
2.   Or double NS** veggies, skip SC*, add one-hundred calories dessert
3.   End with decaf coffee or herbal tea then stop eating
4.   After two hours, enjoy an after-dinner snack:
      one-hundred calories SC* plus one-hundred calories fat

—Avoid SC until dinner or after dinner
—Avoid sugar until dessert except for specified pre-workout drink
—Limit caffeine: two cups per day, then decaf coffee/herbal tea

*SC = Starchy Carbohydrate
**NS = Non-Starchy

Tips

Good Morning, Jesus
- First Five App: Set to your morning alarm, only five minutes!
- You Version Audio Bible App: Listen to the word of God while driving, exercising, etc. (I listen while I spin on the bike.)
- For Those Who Want More: When you read the Bible, listen to an audio version at the same time. This helps with retention!
- Play Worship Music: Equals brighter mornings for everyone.

Breakfast: Enjoy with decaf or regular coffee or tea. Eat after your AM workout. If you do not work out in the AM, just make sure you eat breakfast BEFORE you are tempted by outside junk. DON'T leave home without it!

Lunch: Enjoy with unsweetened tea, decaf green tea, or water with lemon. Lunch/Dinner Chart includes salads with protein and fat. Keep carbs to 15-20 grams and feel free to add shredded carrots or sliced beets. Most people do not include enough lean protein, carbohydrates in the form of veggies, or the right kinds/amounts of fats in their salads. This is why many are starving after a salad! Avoid sugar and bad fats in the form of cranberries (Craisins), candied nuts, sugary dressings, or dressings made with soybean oil. Sugars spike hunger instead of satisfying it. Omega 6 fats in dressings are a health risk. Instead, carry a one-hundred calorie pack of almonds—a better fat than sugary dressings. Or use one tablespoon olive oil and lemon or vinegar as dressing. (Optional: add two tablespoons Greek yogurt to make it creamy. Garlic lovers can also add black garlic, which has a savory flavor.)

Snacks: Enjoy with green, white, or herbal tea. See Breakfast/Snack Chart. A morning snack is optional. If you eat an early lunch, you can move your morning snack to early afternoon and still have an afternoon snack late afternoon. A later afternoon snack is a must! Without it, most people go into dinner starving. This is a recipe for disaster. Starving equals STUFFED.

Pre-Workout Only: Add one tablespoon of honey plus (optional) half teaspoon turmeric to green tea.

Cheese Lovers: Add forty calories to any meal, which is approximately two tablespoons of feta, gorgonzola, parmesan, blue cheese crumbles, cheddar, mozzarella or quarter cup cottage cheese or Greek yogurt.

Chocolate Lovers (anytime): Have a long gap between meals and snacks? Need an afternoon pick me up? Combine one tablespoon coconut butter (not oil) plus half teaspoon raw cacao with hot water and mix well for a delicious hot cacao that curbs hunger (max one per day).

BREAKFAST/SNACK CHART

FAITH VS WEIGHT®

BREAKFAST (Protein/Fat/Fruit)

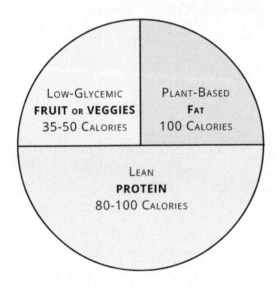

LOW-GLYCEMIC
FRUIT OR VEGGIES
35-50 CALORIES

PLANT-BASED
FAT
100 CALORIES

LEAN
PROTEIN
80-100 CALORIES

BREAKFAST IDEAS (PLATE SHOWN)

Breakfast to Go:

- 1/2 yellow/green banana
- 1/2 cup cottage cheese or 1/2 cup Greek yogurt
- *1 Tbsp nut butter or 2 Tbsp nuts
- Optional: 1 Tbsp ground flax, pinch of salt

Smoothie: Add 1/3 cup water/ice cubes to above and blend (optional: add any leafy green). *Use nut butter instead of nuts if making a smoothie.

For Unlimited Combinations, Substitute:

- Any 1/2 cup low-glycemic fruit or vegetable
- Any nut butter/nuts or plant-based fat for fat
- Any protein: Greek yogurt, eggs/egg whites, bone broth

More Ideas: 2 hard-boiled eggs (eat one yoke) OR 1 hard-boiled egg and 1 light string cheese plus 1 cup raw veggies, 1/4 cup hummus or guacamole OR 1 yellow/green banana with 1 Tbsp peanut butter

Omelet: 1 egg plus 1/4 cup egg whites plus veggies, 1/2 avocado plus 1/2 grapefruit. **Optional:** top omelet with up to 40 calories of cheese (approx. 2 Tbsp cheddar, feta, parmesan, gorgonzola, goat, Colby jack, or mozzarella, etc.). At restaurants, get cheese on the side or just eat half the omelet.

Morning and Afternoon Snack (all plant-based)

Grab and Go:
1. One apple plus 100 calories of almonds or 1 Tbsp almond buter
2. One cup mixed berries plus 100 calories of pistachios
3. Carrots/celery, 100 calories of hummus
4. One six-inch yellow/green banana and one Tbsp peanut butter

(Mix it up: If you had a banana for breakfast, have berries, an apple, or raw veggies for your morning or afternoon snack)

Substitutions:
- Choose any low-glycemic fruit or raw veggies
- Choose any 100-calorie serving of nuts, nut butter, or edamame

(A morning snack is optional, but the afternoon snack is a must!)

If you need a heartier snack than the ones listed, no problem. Just make sure your snack is within the guidelines on the chart (protein, fat, fruit).

Lunch/Dinner Chart

FAITH VS WEIGHT®

Lunch/Dinner (Protein/Fat/Veggies)

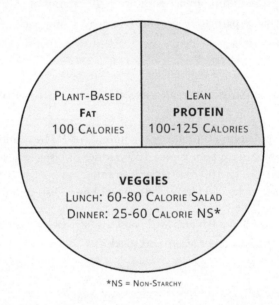

PLANT-BASED
FAT
100 CALORIES

LEAN
PROTEIN
100-125 CALORIES

VEGGIES
LUNCH: 60-80 CALORIE SALAD
DINNER: 25-60 CALORIE NS*

*NS = NON-STARCHY

Lunch Ideas

Protein: 3-4 oz. of grilled chicken, lean meat, fish, lean turkey, shellfish (shrimp, mussels), raw fish (oysters, sashimi, ceviche), 2 hard-boiled eggs (eat only 1 yolk).

Plant-based fats: 100 calories = 1 Tbsp olive oil, 1-2 Tbsp pesto, 1/4 cup hummus, 1/4 cup guacamole. Avoid sugary dressings/sauces.

Salad Greens with Veggies: 2 cups leafy greens with artichokes, beets, tomatoes, carrots, cucumbers, mushrooms, sun-dried tomatoes, etc.
Optional: Add 2 Tbsp beans, chick peas, or peas.

DINNER IDEAS

The Basics: lean protein and plant-based fats listed above. Include non-starchy (NS) veggies: 1 cup of steamed microwaved broccoli, green beans, cauliflower, asparagus, spinach, zucchini, peppers, bok choy, cabbage, summer squash, okra, kale, collard greens, etc.

Less Active

Dinner Only

Add 100 calories of SC (best bets):
- 1/2 medium baked potato
- 1/2 cup sweet potato
- 1/2 cup winter squash
- 1/2 cup corn, peas, or beans
- 1/2 cup any whole grain
- 1/2 cup any whole grain pasta

Add 100 calorie dessert (best bets):
70% dark chocolate, 100 calories of nuts, or 100 calories of skinny pop popcorn

OR Add 200 calories of SC and skip dessert
(End with decaf coffee or tea)

STOP EATING/DRINKING

More Active

Dinner
Add 100 calories of SC, skip dessert
OR Double NS veggies, *Skip SC, Add 100-calorie dessert
(End with decaf coffee or tea)

After Dinner Snack (ADS)
100-calorie SC plus 100-calorie fat

- 3 cups air-popped popcorn with 1 Tbsp light olive oil/salt
- 100-calorie steel-cut oatmeal with 1 Tbsp nut butter/cinnamon

*If you skipped SC at dinner and are very active, you can have up to 200 calories (max) SC as part of your ADS.

STOP EATING/DRINKING

RESTAURANT GUIDE

I always tell my clients I enjoy walking out of a restaurant feeling just as good, if not better, than when I walked in, even when I am on vacation. Why would anybody want to feel worse, especially after spending loads of money? I don't need to feel like Jabba the Hut after the party is over, and neither do you. The only way to do this is to make sure you have an afternoon snack before dinner. If you have a long stretch between breakfast and lunch, you should have a morning snack as well. Showing up to a restaurant at any time of day starving will leave you stuffed.

At every meal, whether you are at a restaurant or at home, you only have three things to think about: lean protein, fat, and veggies. Once you get into the habit of ordering this way, the rest is easy! I have eaten all over the world following this model. If you are at a restaurant that does not have any healthy plant-based fats, you can always have your stash of hundred-calorie nuts at the end of your meal. That counts as your fat. Don't leave home without it! Plant-based fats in the right amounts help flip the switch to beat sugar cravings.

GENERAL TIPS

Decide on your lean protein, plant-based fat, and vegetable options first. *Again, you only have three things to remember.* New clients tell me about meals they were excited about, only to realize they forgot to add a plant-based fat, enough protein, or a vegetable. I have to tell them to eat more next time! Why does this matter? This will affect how hungry you are at the end of the meal, which is a huge issue when the dessert cart rolls around. This will also affect how hungry you are for your next meal or snack. You will either be starving from eating too little (trying to be virtuous) or starving at the end of your sugar roller-coaster ride from overdoing dessert. Sound familiar? Since you crave what you eat, overdoing sugar leads to overdoing more sugar. This same caution goes toward forgetting or ignoring the advice to eat a FAITH VS. WEIGHT breakfast and an afternoon snack. Failing to do so will set you up for failure. See the breakfast/ snack chart. This plan makes snacks so easy you only need to pick *two ingredients* as you walk out the door!

Problems arise when you try to beat the system. "If I skip the fat, then I can have more dessert." Brilliant! It all sounds great until you realize you have taken in considerably more calories at dessert than you would have if you had just included the plant-based fat in the first place. The same goes for skipping breakfast or the afternoon snacks on this plan, thinking you will spend those same calories on dessert. This never happens. People always overdo it. Others skip meals/snacks because they think this will lead to faster weight loss. If either of these cases were true, there would not be an obesity epidemic. Occasionally, when I ask a client why she did not include enough vegetables and her hundred calories of plant-based fat, she will tell me, "Well, I was just not that hungry." This makes logical sense. However, later today or tomorrow, she is starving. Your body concludes it did not get enough calories, so it must be time to *go for it* the next time you start eating! Skipping a meal/snack or part of one is the equivalent of being what I like to call *penny wise and pounds foolish*, which is exactly why most diets fail.

Portion Sizes

At all meals, especially at restaurants, your number one priority is portion sizes. The easiest way to keep portion sizes in check at restaurants is to ask for a separate plate. Serve yourself the correct size portions from your entrée plate onto this separate plate. Decide the amount you are going to eat *before* you start eating. Once you start talking, your attention starts walking. Many start out with good intentions, thinking they will just eat half, but this is hit or miss. Putting the right amounts on a separate plate makes it easier. You can share the rest or take it home.

Prudence is making the decision of how much you are going to eat *before you eat it.*

Your future should not be left in the hands of the overworked cook in the back since they are not going to drive you to your doctor or pay for your meds.

The best way to guesstimate serving size amounts at home or at a restaurant is the following:

Protein: Palm-size portion of fish, shellfish, lean meat, lean poultry, or cooked egg (stick with egg whites, or one egg with one egg white). Enjoy your proteins grilled, baked, or raw (in the case of sashimi or ceviche).

Dairy: If you enjoy cheese, always ask for it on the side. If someone else adds it, it will most likely be double the amount. Once it is on the side, you can then add up to forty to fifty calories to your meal, which roughly comes to two tablespoons of feta, shredded Parmesan, gorgonzola, or blue cheese crumbles (which is different from blue cheese dressing). You are much better off with real blue cheese crumbles than sugary or cheap oil dressings. If you prefer plain yogurt or cottage cheese, you can add up to one-quarter cup. If you are having an omelet already prepared with cheese, eat half of it, since most restaurants tend to overdo cheese.

The only time to have half a cup of yogurt or cottage cheese is if that is your only protein. For example, you may grab a cottage cheese and a banana with a few nuts. In that case, have a half cup.

Fat: Always ask for all nuts, oils, pesto, guacamole, and hummus on the side. Almost every time fat is added ahead of time, excess is added. Many times I have seen well-meaning people order an egg white omelet, only to receive it drenched in oil. You can bet the oil was not heart healthy, and the amount was hundreds of calories more than what is recommended on this plan. I always ask for my omelets to be prepared "dry" or with minimal oil if they are unable to cook it dry. Then I have my fats on the side. Avocado is a delicious complement to any omelet. Serving sizes of fats are one tablespoon of olive oil, two tablespoons nuts, two tablespoons pesto, one half sliced avocado, one-fourth cup guacamole or hummus. If you are not sure what a one-fourth cup looks like, just remember a one-fourth cup equals four tablespoons. For guacamole or hummus, you can get a small dish and spoon out four level tablespoons instead of continually digging into a huge bowl and losing track. Avoid candied nuts and sugary dressings. If you get dressings/sauces on the side, dip your fork in first and *then* pick up your food. If you do it the other way around, you will take in hundreds more calories. Adding one tablespoon of extra virgin olive oil is a much better choice than any commercially produced salad dressing or sauce. If you prefer nuts and olive oil, you can mix it up with two teaspoons of olive oil and one tablespoon of nuts.

Veggies: At lunch, enjoy an entrée-size salad of any type of greens with tomatoes, cucumbers, artichokes, mushrooms, and so on. Add a few starchy veggies like sliced beets or carrots and no more than two tablespoons of chickpeas, beans, or peas, keeping total carbohydrate to fifteen to twenty grams.

At dinner, always enjoy water with lime or lemon when you sit down. Remember the suggestion to order a salad or raw veggies with some healthy fat like guacamole, olives, or olive oil as a salad dressing as your appetizer. If not, you will be starving by the time your entrée comes because everyone else will have ordered an appetizer. Even if you order a FAITH VS. WEIGHT meal, you are more likely to get off track because starving equals stuffed, which may result in you face-planting into the nachos before your entrée is even out of the oven.

With regard to your entrée, enjoy a lean protein. Then fill at least half of your plate with non-starchy veggies. Since you have the option to include a starchy carbohydrate at dinner or after dinner, depending on your activity level, it makes sense to keep the veggies on the non-starchy side. You can add fats to your entrée as listed on the lunch/dinner chart. If you have already had a fat with your appetizer, keep that in mind.

Timing of Starchy Carbohydrates

These are enjoyed at dinner or after dinner only (see eating timing and tips). Skip them before dinner, unless you are adding the starchy veggies listed for lunch. The kicker is you don't always have healthy starchy carb options available (see lunch/dinner chart) when you are out to eat. This means you have a decision to make. You can have your starchy carb calories at dinner or save them as an after-dinner option. If you are not in a rush to lose weight, you can have whatever starchy carb at the restaurant you want as long as it does not exceed one hundred calories of carbohydrate. In order to be able to succeed at this, it is *highly recommended* that you eat your protein or veggies *first*. If you start out with the bread basket or nachos, it's all downhill from there, and most people just keep on going. This doesn't mean you cannot have any. *It does mean* getting a small plate and then putting it aside until the end of the meal. Sip your water with lemon or lime or eat the side salad you ordered as an appetizer. Again, eat your protein or veggies first.

View your carb almost as a dessert, because that is pretty much how your body is viewing it. If you want to save a roll with a pat of butter for the end, then go for it. More is not better. Your starchy carbohydrate on this plan equals one medium size roll, a one half cup of pasta or rice, or half of a medium-sized baked or sweet potato. A small fist size of winter squash is a great choice. If you have never been able to stop at one serving with starchy carbs, you may think this impossible. This is where eating your protein and veggies first comes in handy. Eating your carbohydrates with fat *last* can make all the difference.

Desserts

(See eating timing and tips.) The most common pitfall with desserts at restaurants is what I call the *community trough*. This is where a dessert (or two or three) is ordered for the group, and everyone keeps sticking their fork in until it is all gone. We have all been there! This winds up being a race you will never win. We are not only overdoing unhealthy fats, we are combining them with loads of sugar before the dinner plates have even been cleared.

Instead, ask for a dessert plate and put a small serving (usually the size of two thumbs) on it. Order a decaf coffee or herbal tea and savor your dessert as you play the game to see how long it will last. More is not better. In fact, people are less satisfied when they overdo it. Happy faces are not what I see when the party is over. Eat it slowly. If you race to eat your dessert, I promise you will lose, and it will not be weight.

More about Protein

When it comes to protein, fish is a personal preference. However, I am also biased to the fact that people seem to lose weight faster and keep it off easier when they eat more fish. Maybe it has something to do with those omega-3s. If you are lucky enough to be at a restaurant that serves wild-caught salmon, that is my first choice over other animal proteins. Of course, shrimp or oysters are always a treat. Occasionally you may be fortunate enough to find grass-fed beef or free-range chicken.

Finally, remind yourself that you can eat as much as you want as often as you want as long as you want, if that's what you really want. I have a sign on my desk that says, "If you feel like quitting, remember why you started in the first place."

RESTAURANT OPTIONS

Pray before your meals.

TWO THINGS TO REMEMBER:

1. Order a salad with olive oil as an appetizer when with a group, or raw veggies with a healthy fat, so you are not tempted to eat hundreds of calories before your meal even arrives because the table has ordered a high-calorie bomb.

2. You can have your starchy carbohydrate serving at the restaurant or you can skip the starchy carb at dinner and save it for home or later for your after-dinner snack, depending on your activity level. If you skip a starchy carbohydrate at dinner, remember to double your serving of vegetables. Don't forget to add a healthy fat. Then you can still have a *small* dessert with an herbal tea or decaf coffee.

Mediterranean

*Protein: chicken or shrimp kabob (lamb on occasion)

Veggie: fattoush salad (cucumber garden salad)

Fat: quarter cup hummus baba ghanoush (ask for raw vegetables for dipping)

*Some have good bean dishes (fava, lentil … just keep to quarter cup when having it with other proteins)

Possible Dinner Starchy Carb Options:

1. Half cup brown rice
2. Half whole grain pita bread (if you are lucky, you may find gluten-free)
3. Half pita bread or half cup rice

Mexican

Protein: grilled fajitas: shrimp, chicken, or beef with black beans

Veggie: salad or peppers/onions

Fat: quarter cup guacamole

Optional Condiment: salsa

Possible Dinner Starchy Carb Options:

1. Half cup brown rice
2. Two small corn or one medium flour tortilla
3. If you have a hankering for chips, count out about twelve to fourteen and separate them onto a plate to eat with your meal so you don't keep going and going. Have them with a healthy fat like a quarter cup guacamole, after you eat your protein and vegetables. (Avoid chips at the start since this tends to lead to mindless eating.)

GREEK

*Protein: chicken gyro meat (lamb on occasion)

Veggie: Greek salad (ask for dressing and feta on the side)

Fat: hummus or baba ghanoush (one quarter cup)

(ask for raw vegetables for dipping and skip the pita bread)

Condiment: can add one to two tablespoons of feta

* Some have good bean dishes (fava, lentil ... just keep to quarter cup when having it with other proteins)

Possible Dinner Starchy Carb Options:

1. Half cup brown rice
2. Half whole grain pita bread (if you are lucky, you may find gluten-free)
3. Half pita bread or half cup rice

CHINESE

*Protein and veggie: steamed vegetables with shrimp or chicken breast are your best options. (Steamed shrimp and broccoli are my favorites.)

Fat: I usually scan the menu for a sauce that looks good, one without sugar (e.g., sesame oil on the side), or have almonds on the side (two tablespoons).

*Some have black beans as an option. Keep to a quarter cup when having it with other proteins.

Possible Dinner Starchy Carb Options:

1. Half cup brown or white rice (brown is best)
2. Half cup soba or noodles

JAPANESE

*Protein: salmon sashimi (no rice) or grilled fish/chicken

Condiment: ginger or wasabi (both are great)

Condiment: lite soy sauce

Veggie: salad with dressing on the side

Fat: side of avocado (they will bring you sliced avocado), max one-half medium avocado

Tip: miso soup (high in sodium but broth soups help cut caloric intake)

Unless you are at a fancy Japanese restaurant, most seaweed salads are loaded with sugar.

*Edamame or black beans as an option (keep to quarter cup when having it with other proteins)

Possible Dinner Starchy Only Carb Options:

1. Half cup brown or white rice (brown is best)
2. Half cup soba or noodles

ITALIAN

*Protein: grilled fish or chicken (Macaroni Grill has a fabulous shrimp scallop dish with garlic over steamed spinach. Add one tablespoon of Parmesan to taste if preferred.)

Veggies: spinach, broccoli, peppers (ask for them steamed) or salad

Fat: one to two tablespoons pesto, olives (on the side - two tablespoons), or one tablespoon olive oil)

*One cup of lentil soup can be added as part of your protein serving.

Possible Dinner Starchy Carb Options:

1.　Half cup roasted potatoes
2.　Half cup pasta (Macaroni Grill has whole wheat and gluten-free pasta.)

AMERICAN

*Protein: grilled fish or chicken

Veggie: salad with dressing on the side or steamed veggies

Fat:　two tablespoons of nuts or olives; one-half avocado; or quarter cup of guacamole or hummus

Skip the dried fruit.

Fat: dressing on the side

*Chili is an option. Keep it to one cup.

Possible Dinner Starchy Carb Options:

1.　Half cup brown or white rice (brown is best)
2.　Half cup pasta (whole grain or gluten free is best)
3.　Half cup quinoa or other ancient grains
4.　Half cup corn or peas
5.　Small baked or sweet potato

Pancake Houses/ Brunch

*Protein: dry egg white omelet (Dry is made without oil. In this case, they usually use Pam. You may need to say no oil.)

Veggie: extra spinach and veggies for the omelet (Tabasco if you like it)

Condiment: Salsa is okay. Tip: I ask for Parmesan on the side and add two tablespoons to my omelet.

Fat: half a sliced avocado

Pancake House/Dinner

Possible Dinner Only Carb Options:

1. Yes you can have dinner for breakfast! I order whole grain pancakes as my favorite dinner for breakfast carb, and spread peanut butter on the pancake.
2. Half a cup steel-cut oatmeal. You can add one tablespoon nut butter with cinnamon.

Fast Food

Protein: grilled chicken salad

Fat: dressing on the side

Fat: (Add one hundred calories of pistachios if desired.)

Specific Restaurants

Ci Ci's: You can order the salad bar and ask for chicken, and they will bring it from the back. You can also ask for olives. Make sure you have your regular snacks before entering the world of pizza. (You can get olives for your healthy fat here.)

Fuddruckers: You can order the salmon sandwich, garden salad, and a side of avocado. You can get rid of the bun and throw the salmon on the salad with the avocado.

Subway: You can get the chopped salad and order every vegetable they have. Choose the grilled chicken and get a side of guacamole for the dressing. (Their whole grain breads are more dough than grain).

Starbucks: For drinks, green, hibiscus, mint tea, or coffee, decaf coffee black (you can add cinnamon). For breakfast or lunch, egg white bites or protein plate are great choices. They also carry unsweetened almond butter. If you are lucky, you may even find a green banana.

FAITH VS. WEIGHT

Testimonials

My name is Pat, and I stand here today humble and thankful for my life. I have decided to share my story with you. My family has a high rate of obesity, and I thought that there would never be anything that I could do about my weight. I struggled most of my life with dieting and weight, and it became harder after having children. If you can name at least five to ten diets, I probably have tried them all, with no success or a small temporary fix.

In 2007, I shattered both of my legs in a terrible fall and was wheelchair bound for three and a half years. I was told that I was never going to walk again. In 2009, I became a single parent taking care of my three special needs boys. After years of rehab, I was able to walk again.

God obviously had other plans for me …

I decided to join the YMCA, where I met Maria Bower. Little did I know that Maria was watching me. She approached me on several occasions and told me I was working out too long and not getting results. She also told me that 80 percent of losing weight was nutrition. So I decided to try her concept of FAITH VS. WEIGHT. I did not expect to have a drastic change in my weight. But it happened (not just for me but for others at the YMCA), and it is real. Over the last year, following Maria's FAITH VS. WEIGHT program, I have totally changed my life. I have lost over fifty pounds.

The concept is very easy, and she incorporates foods that you enjoy into your daily life. We are all given gifts from God, and this is Maria's calling. Please, do not let her pass you by. Try her out, and she will change your life forever. Her concepts on how nutrition and weight loss work will never leave you.

Thank you, Maria … Thank you.

—Pat K.
(lost seventy pounds)

I was a participant in the FAITH VS. WEIGHT program about six months ago. As a longtime Weight Watchers member and regular exerciser, I was interested to see what more I could learn through this program. Maria has unbelievable energy, enthusiasm, and knowledge of weight management and healthy eating. I learned the importance of portion control, that I can have a small treat every day, and that God truly cares about my weight and how it relates to my health. In the past six months, I've lost fifteen pounds and gone from a size 4 to a size 2. FAITH VS. WEIGHT is supportive and educational: a great way to get control of your eating habits.

—Gayle W.

I lost a total of eleven pounds during your seven-week class. At first, I thought I must have a dreadful disease because never, ever, ever has weight loss come that easy for me. Every week I would come in and say that I wasn't following the program as well as I should, but evidently you were getting in my brain, and I must have been making some small changes that were good.

—Becky R.

FAITH VS. WEIGHT has been a successful combination of inspiration and information for my husband and I. Over the years, we have tried to eat healthier and lose weight by using quick-fix options like fad diets, fasting, Jenny Craig, and Weight Watchers, but we didn't really know what being healthy meant. By following the FAITH VS. WEIGHT lifestyle, we have lost over sixty-five pounds in the last six months! Through this program, we have learned to integrate our faith into our lifestyle choices, helping us to start a healthier chapter in our lives! FAITH VS. WEIGHT has inspired to us to not only eat better but to live better.

—Sarah E.

I have tried so many plans, including Weight Watchers, which did not work at all for me. I have bought every magazine that promises instant weight loss. I have a library full of books on every diet plan. Maria made a big difference because she made the plan personal to my needs and was willing to change and add to the plan for each individual. That makes a huge difference. Also, it was so easy to follow. I do not feel deprived and do not miss sugar. I never ate fat but now am adding avocado, olives, and olive oil and am amazed at how the cravings for sugary foods has gone away. As a diabetic, I do have to count carbs, but for the non-diabetic, there is really no counting. I have found I can easily follow this when I go out to eat and was so surprised to find that I did not feel deprived. The idea of ordering a salad when everyone else has appetizers works great for me. I also do what Maria suggests about asking for a take-home plate, and then I am not temped to continue eating when I am content. The drop in insulin really got me going and is keeping me on the plan. I am not craving junk food, and by eating four times a day (which is what diabetics are supposed to do), I can manage my hunger and what I eat much better. *I have stopped grazing.* Maria encouraged us to take baby steps and just try to set and reach a new goal each week. That is so helpful. This plan is something I can continue and really takes very little effort.

—Linda R. (For more of Linda's testimony, check out
"A Day in the Life of a Diabetic.")

Maria included scripture in every class, and I was impressed by the amount of biblical knowledge that she had. She blended together scripture, prayer, Bible stories, and cutting-edge knowledge about the science of different foods and how each individual body processes them as well as how exercise for each person's body type improves body function, weight loss, and energy. Her main goal was for us to learn to eat properly and have a healthy, fit body in order to have energy to work for the kingdom of God. The healthy part includes prevention (which should start at an early age), control of major diseases such as heart disease, diabetes, osteoporosis, and other things that come with aging. This causes people to visit the doctor or be in the hospital, preventing them from serving Jesus. She also included tips for foods for growing kids, since she has two middle-school-aged boys.

The class format each week included opening prayer, scripture verses, a virtue of the week (prudence, temperance, justice, faith, etc.), an action plan for the week, and sharing our joys and concerns for how we were doing. At the beginning of the class, we were challenged to come up with a mantra and a verse for our seven-week journey to healthy eating and weight loss. Mine was, "Today is the first day of the rest of my life," and the scripture was Philippians 3:13–14. Each week, our homework included writing a nightly letter to God and a challenge of things to do for your body and for your spirit each day.

I definitely saw success in my eating patterns, weight loss (don't have any scales but lost two pant sizes!), daily exercise, and have so much more energy for the things I'm doing to serve the Lord. Art and I are going to Romania this summer on a mission trip, and part of my motivation for taking this class was to get in good physical shape to be able to serve to the best of my ability as well as each week in choir. Also, I want to stay healthy and fit for as long as possible.

Another class member was going through a divorce, has MS, and was struggling with her weight. She was able to lose fifteen pounds, and we were blessed to be able to pray with her through her struggles with the divorce and her job search. Other class members had issues with being addicted to sugar and were able to learn methods to prevent their addiction from taking control, and some were at a plateau in their weight loss and received valuable tips to help their weight-loss battle. Amazing things happen when we eat like God intended!

All these negative things happen because the enemy is so determined to thwart our ability to live a victorious life in Jesus, and through prayer, scripture, and group support, we are able to overcome and win the battle. If we are victims to our eating habits and disease, we cannot be warriors for Christ. Thanks again for promoting the class. It (and God) have definitely changed my life. Love you!

—Joanie R.

`I can't wait to tell you this news. I am twenty pounds lighter! I don't think any weight loss occurred before I joined your class. I never told anyone this, but at my last physical, my doctor said I was almost pre-diabetic. It still took me till October to do anything about it. Your program has saved me! All my levels are down! I lowered my cholesterol from 198 to126. All my levels are completely normal! I have always been on cholesterol medication because my liver just produces too much. One twenty-six is a great number for me. Thank you for your inspiration and wisdom. I'm able to serve the kingdom better because of you! I am beyond happy. I can't even describe the joy I am feeling from inside! God is so good! Praise, praise, praise!

—Jess A.

I wanted to let you know how much I enjoyed the FAITH VS. WEIGHT program. Being inspired by God, Maria Bower created this program as she lovingly recognized a need in our community because so many people are dealing with unhealthy eating issues. Weekly, she shared a virtue from God's Word and applicable Bible verses, encouraging her students to trust God for everything, including our eating challenges. She has done numerous hours of research to find the best healthy eating plan. Maria offered her students a list of food choices to make shopping easier and developed simplified meal plans, giving the students the tools to healthy living. Maria's nonjudgmental attitude made it comfortable for students to share their personal concerns about specific food choices or eating issues. She always offered invaluable advice and suggestions. Maria was sympathetic to the demands of women especially and shared quick, healthy meal options for the on-the-go woman. She also shared exercise tips for specific body types. I would highly recommend this program to any man or woman who wants to feel healthy and to live a happy and fulfilled life that God so truly wants for each of us. I am blessed to have met Maria and am so grateful for all the information and knowledge that she shared with all of us.

—Debbie H.

Impressions from program ...

> "Coming together to pray, discuss fears, and celebrate triumphs is a must."

> "Just the right amount of faith, diet, and exercise material."

> "My prayer now is that God, not food, will fill the empty place in my heart."

When asked what was most valuable about the program ...

> "Nutrition and exercise information."

> "The spiritual affirmation."

> "The open-forum ability to ask questions."

> "Teacher enthusiasm and expertise."

When asked if participants would recommend the FAITH VS. WEIGHT program to a friend or church group ...

> "Yes, I already did."

> "One hundred percent yes!"

> "Absolutely!"

> Check out mariabower.com for additional testimonials and class offerings.

A Day in the Life
of a Diabetic (Q&A)

With Linda R.

1. How has the FAITH VS. WEIGHT plan made a difference for you as a diabetic?

During the six weeks I attended the class, I dropped from thirty-six units of Lantus at night to twenty-eight units. This is huge. I have lost eight pounds. I was at a low in my diabetes management before taking this class. I knew exactly what to do but just wasn't doing it. My diabetic educator said this is a very common thing with longtime diabetics. I had just lost my energy to manage it daily (and it does take energy). The class helped me get back on track. The meal plans offered were easy to remember and were like the one I had received from my education class. I am now back to exercising, which makes a huge difference in blood sugar control (fifteen to twenty minutes after each meal when I can). My before-meal insulin has dropped from eight to ten units to five to six, depending on carb intake and amount of exercise and pre-meal readings. These are huge drops in insulin, and my doctor is so pleased. Besides dropping insulin, the readings are so much better. It is almost impossible to be successful with diabetes management without counting carbs. This plan has helped me get back to eating healthy fats, which helps a lot with cravings. Also, diabetics are supposed to supplement meals with healthy low-carb snacks, and this plan has helped me get back on track. The plan has also helped me to change the carb intake for breakfast and lunch, resulting in better readings.

2. Describe a typical day of eating. How have you modified this plan?

The number one thing that has helped me is to sit down and eat and not eat on the go! Before this plan, I was not good about eating breakfast. I am still not a big breakfast eater but try to stay with one of the choices from the plan every day. (I also add juice from half a lemon to my early-morning decaf tea.) I eat eggs for breakfast. I love to add veggies and scramble them together. I also have Canadian bacon, a piece of whole grain forty-five-calorie toast with avocado and tomatoes or whole grain toast with nut butter. I use low-carb forty-five-calorie bread and do not have that every morning. I like to add a small mandarin orange. For lunch, I have started eating more salads and veggies. I love salads and make dressing out of olive oil or pecan oil and flavored vinegars. My protein is usually chicken, sometimes a little lean beef, and every now and then a small amount of cheese. My snack is usually an apple and a cheese stick or nut butter. That is easy, and I love it. Dinner is light. I follow the plan as closely as I can, and I usually test as soon as I get up and take my Metformin. I have found that doing this, my liver stops putting out sugar, and my breakfast reading will be good. If the sugar gets out of hand in the early morning, it is almost impossible to get it under control for the whole day.

So many people are walking around and don't even know they are diabetic or pre-diabetic.

(Check out the rest of Linda's experience in the testimonials section of this book.)

About the Author

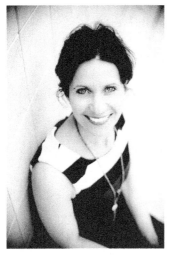

MARIA BOWER is a Born Again Christian who is blessed to be surrounded by her favorite people in the whole wide world. In order to fully recognize and appreciate this, she makes it a top priority to start each new day abiding in the Lord and spending time beholding His glory. As the wife of an active husband and mother of very busy middle and high school aged boys, she needs all of the energy she can get, while also keeping up with their two Australian shepherds, Summer and Winter. Her morning time with the Lord also energizes her for the pre-destined opportunities that inevitably come her way to spread the Gospel, whether it is through volunteering, grocery shopping, or getting a haircut. Maria prays for boldness before, during, and after each encounter, especially when it would honestly be easier to keep her mouth shut and focus on the latest celebrity gossip at the checkout stand or salon.

Her active hobbies include swimming, jogging, walking, cycling, boxing, shooting (she does live in Texas), and teaching exercise classes. Her more relaxing hobbies include either reading books or listening to audio versions of books. Although she loves to read, she hates to sit, so even reading is accomplished during some form of movement. To most, she appears to be very busy, but somehow she still manages to find the time to frequent her local

Hobby Lobby, insisting that they might put out a missing person's report if she misses her biweekly visits. Because of her penchant for framed biblical quotes, she is currently running out of wall space in her office.

Maria loves to teach the seven-week FAITH VS. WEIGHT program that this book is based on at Prestonwood Baptist Church in Plano, Texas, and is absolutely thrilled whenever she has the opportunity through speaking engagements to get people more excited about having more energy to serve the kingdom.

To find out more about Maria's classes; follow her on social media; or read her occasional blogs at mariabower.com

To share your testimonials, contact maria@faithvsweight.com

To book a speaking engagement, please contact maria@faithvsweight.com

Your comments are welcome! Please review this book on Amazon.

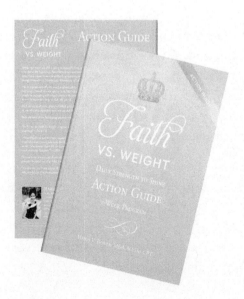

Purchase the

Faith Vs. Weight
Daily Strength to Shine
Action Guide
7-Week Program

for additional support.

Available at Amazon and other online retailers.

Made in the USA
Coppell, TX
10 February 2022

73299633R00225